This Book Will Make You Feel Something

SPHERE

First published in Great Britain in 2023 by Sphere

1 3 5 7 9 10 8 6 4 2

A CIP catalogue record for this book
is available from the British Library.

Trade paperback ISBN: 978-1-4087-2840-6

Designed and typeset in Mrs Eaves and Brandon Grotesque by HART STUDIO
Printed and bound in China by C & C Offset Printing Co Ltd

Papers used by Sphere are from well-managed forests
and other responsible sources.

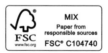

Sphere
An imprint of
Little, Brown Book Group
Carmelite House
50 Victoria Embankment
London EC4Y 0DZ

An Hachette UK Company
www.hachette.co.uk

www.littlebrown.co.uk

This Book Will Make You Feel Something

Masturbation meditations
to enjoy on your own or
with a partner

Florence Bark

SPHERE

CONTENTS

INTRODUCTION

It feels like I spent most of my youth masturbating. I remember the exact moment I first discovered that touching myself felt good, and from that day everything changed. I was finding objects that vibrated everywhere – my mouse toy, which 'ran' across surfaces with pulsing vibrations; the wiggle pen that vibrated so that it made your writing go all curly; my Nokia brick phone; the PlayStation controller – and I've never stopped. I love masturbating. I hope you love it, too. I hope you feel proud enough to bring it up in conversations, to say you can't go for dinner because you have plans with your vibrator, to discuss with friends how you like to do it, to ask them what they think about when *they're* doing it. But the truth is, there's a good chance you don't do any of the above. We all know someone who kept their teenage masturbation habits secret – I did too, to a degree – and, combined with various other cultural reasons, that shame has pervaded into our feelings about it as adults. One recent survey suggested as many as 53 per cent of us feel uncomfortable talking about masturbation, despite 91 per cent of women doing it.[1] With this book, I'm on a mission to change that, and there are several very good reasons why that change is important.

Before I tell you what they are, let me introduce myself. My name is Florence Bark; I've been working in the sex education, relationship and intimacy space for a decade. I'm the co-presenter of ComeCurious, a YouTube platform I created in 2015 with my bestie, Reed Amber. We also started a podcast so that we could talk even more about sex, as if that was even possible, a now award-winning little number called F**ks Given. Everything we do has been about starting the conversation around sex in hopes that we can battle the shame and stigmas surrounding pleasure and help everybody to have the best sex life possible.

So, why is female masturbation so important that I've written a whole book to encourage you to do it?

1. It feels good. Anything that feels good is important.

2. It's self-care – and don't let anybody tell you otherwise. Taking half an hour, or a whole evening, or even just ten minutes, to disappear into your mind and appreciate how powerful you are – that it's *you* creating all that pleasure – can only be a great thing. More than that, it's scientifically proven to have benefits for your brain. Masturbation and orgasm helps to release endorphins, oxytocin, serotonin and dopamine – the happy hormones. In a nutshell? It's a happiness booster and stress reliever. That's why I'm referring to the erotica in this book as 'masturbation meditations' – it's because I take the power of masturbation seriously, and I want everybody else to, too.

3. It can help your external sex life. I say 'external', because masturbation *is* a sex life in my opinion. But should you happen to be having sex with a partner or partners, then masturbation can help you to figure out what you want them to be doing to you to increase your chances of orgasm during sex. I'm adamant about this one because research into how many people orgasm during sex routinely puts women at the bottom of the pile, with the biggest orgasm gap existing between straight men and straight women. One survey I've seen on British men and women found 61 per cent of straight men cum during sex compared to 30 per cent of straight women[2]; another on US college students found 91 per cent of straight men cum compared to 39 per cent of straight women – that's a huge 52 per cent gap. Orgasm doesn't need to be the goal every time you have sex, of course, but personally I find those

statistics pretty unfair. What's the solution? Well, research tells us only around 30 per cent of women can cum through penetration on its own. The rest of us need clitoral stimulation[3]. If roughly 30 per cent of straight women are saying they cum routinely during sex and roughly only 30 per cent can cum through penetration alone, I think we can safely assume that our great friend the clitoris is being left out of the equation too much of the time. That's perhaps not surprising when you consider porn and the sex scenes in movies and TV shows make it look as if penetration is all we need to orgasm. I'd love it if we all made the clitoris the queen not just during masturbation or foreplay, but during penetrative sex as well. I hope this book will help you to really admire the wonders your clitoris can create, and then you can tell your partner all about it.

4. It can make you feel more confident about your body. If you already masturbate and it's never made you feel better about yours, please don't start wondering if you've been doing it wrong. The trick is that we need to lean into that side of masturbation's benefits and probably nothing else out there in our culture has been encouraging you to do that. Never fear, this book is here! I'm going to do my best through the tips in this book to help you to feel great about you.

So what will you find in this book? Twenty-five electric tips on how to make the most out of masturbation and twenty-five erotic stories to titillate your mind. The stories are here because, as you may already know, arousal starts in your head. We need something sexy to get us turned on that we can obsess over while we're playing with ourselves. While some women do watch porn (and increasingly so), others have reasons for disliking it, and one of those reasons is that the women onscreen might not look like them, or their lovers might not look like how they want them to look. By reading these masturbation meditations rather than watching them, you can put your own stamp of imagination on them and ensure they get you going in a way that works best for you. I've purposely left details about the characters to a minimum so you can do this.

I've included the tips because firstly, I don't believe we're properly taught about our anatomy at school to fully understand how to make the most of it; secondly, to help you explore and get intimate with your body and find out what you like; and thirdly, to shake up your routine and help you get the most out of masturbation's incredible possibilities.

A caveat before we continue: I am a cis woman and have been straight facing most of my life; I am heavily, deeply attracted to men, so even though I now identify as bisexual, the stories in this book reflect my own desires and are probably mostly going to appeal to straight, bi or pan women. That doesn't mean it's just MF (male–female) arrangements in the stories – even if we only want to sleep with people of another gender in real life, we often still want to fantasise about our own; it's actually very common and totally hot. Regardless of my own identity, everyone is welcome to the party, so slip in deep with me and let me know what you think! You will find that some of the tips are written specifically for vulva owners – so if you have other genitals it will be interesting revision for potential partners, or fun facts that I hope you'll find eye-opening. I am also an able-bodied person; if you're not then I hope everything in this book is still helpful to you, but be aware you might need to adapt some of the tips to suit your needs.

Finally, before we get into the juicy bits, I want you to redefine masturbation. While masturbation is a perfectly amazing word and activity, it doesn't encompass the whole experience that we have with ourselves when we are enjoying solo pleasure. I would encourage you to think of it as solo sex. Not having to rely on a partner to feel intimacy, and feeling the magic that touching ourselves can bring – that deserves more noise. If we're having solo sex, then we're having sex by ourselves as independent women and people – that's just as much something to talk about, rave about and make time for as sex with somebody else.

Next time you're masturbating (maybe when you read the first story . . .) give it a go: think of it as solo sex – you having sex with yourself. And, for the record, I bet you're much better at it and bring yourself way more pleasure than most of the people you've slept with. So celebrate yourself.

RECOMMENDATIONS ON HOW TO USE THIS BOOK

If you want to read it cover to cover, be my guest! Though personally I would suggest you start with the Top Tip on page 14 (as I hope it'll help you throughout the whole book) and then pick a masturbation meditation based on what kind of fantasy would most turn you on today. To help with this, you'll find a key at the start of each meditation letting you know what you can expect. You can also try out the flow chart on pages 20 and 21 to help you narrow down what you'd most like to immerse yourself in each time you pick the book up.

Each meditation is preceded by a tip, and while you can skip over it, I'd encourage you to give it a read – it might give you an idea that will blow your mind! If you find you keep returning to a handful of the same stories, pick a different tip from before another story so you can keep expanding your knowledge.

You might want to read the story through once and then masturbate, or you might want to masturbate as you read – we've designed the book so that once you've cracked the spine it should stay open on the page you're looking at. However you do it, I'd definitely suggest you read as slowly as possible. Hold each word in your mouth and swirl your tongue over it – maybe even read it aloud to yourself. When we're turned on we can get the urge to rush ahead, but I would really encourage you to savour the experience and allow yourself to sink into the moment. But also, do exactly what you want to do – you know how you like it!

You'll notice that towards the very end of each meditation there's a line or two in bold. This is the climax of the characters. I've done this so that if you would like to time your orgasm to coincide with the orgasm in the story, then you can glance ahead to see roughly how far away you are from it.

If you have a partner, why not ask them to join you for one or two? Maybe you could even get them to read the tip and then they can do whatever it recommends, if relevant, while you sit back and read the story out loud.

Once you've finished this book – or even while you're reading it – *talk* about it. We all need to talk more about female masturbation with friends and family. In the 1970s, a feminist called Nancy Friday published *My Secret Garden: Women's Sexual Fantasies*, and another sexual revolutionary, Betty Dodson, published a seminal tome called *Sex for One: The Joy of Self-Loving*. Those books were bestsellers and were supposed to change everything. Five decades on and women still struggle to articulate what turns them on and to give masturbation the priority it deserves. There are many cultural reasons as to why and they could take up a whole book on their own. I'd rather you masturbate so let's not get stuck on that, but the point is: it's in our power to change all this. Start talking! But go touch yourself first.

NOTES ON YOUR
MASTURBATION MEDITATIONS

I'm going to be referring to our genitals with certain words that I personally think are some of the sexiest words in the dictionary. My go-to for the vulva and vagina is PUSSY. I'm writing that in capitals for dramatic effect and efficiency in getting to know the word. It's sexy, it's elegant, it's perfect. My go-to for the penis is COCK; for example, *I grab his rock-hard cock and . . .* There is something about the word cock that just feels seductive coming out of your mouth. I highly recommend saying these words out loud a few times just for fun.

For the avoidance of doubt between 'come over here' and 'I want you to cum now', I have spelled the version that involves orgasm or ejaculation as 'cum' throughout. Teenage me would be so proud of this.

How long you want to masturbate for is entirely up to you and I'm personally up for a good hour-long session every now and then! But as research suggests that women on average spend five to ten minutes on one orgasm when touching themselves[4] (it's longer when you have sex), the stories all roughly take five to ten minutes to read. You can, of course, read more than one in a single session.

All the characters in these stories have given their full consent to have sex. I'm saying that so you don't need to let your mind start worrying about that when you're reading – these are fantasies, so allow yourself to get lost in them. I'm also saying that so everyone remembers that consent in sex is very important – *your* consent is essential and don't ever forget it.

Maybe there are some things in here which will give you ideas for your own sex life, but please don't take any of it as instructions and remember that certain things – having sex in a park or against an alleyway wall, for example – are illegal.

THE TOP TIP: GET TO KNOW YOUR ANATOMY

The Collins dictionary defines masturbation as:

**'The stimulation or manipulation of one's
own genitals, esp. to orgasm'**

Sexy, huh? This definition leaves out arguably the most important part of masturbation: the brain. You can touch yourself silly, but if you're not in the mood then you'll likely feel almost nothing. That's a very big topic and something I'll be discussing on page 22, but for my 'top' tip we're going to concentrate on the genitals. Masturbation can be amazing even if we don't orgasm (more on that later, too), but if we do want to have one, or just want to experience more pleasure, then we need to properly understand what we're working with down there: the where, the what and the why.

To do this, I want you to get a mirror, find somewhere nice, warm and comfy to sit, drop your pants and open your legs. Even if you know all this stuff already – go on, indulge me. I have purposely not included a diagram because I want you to be your own diagram. (Though I highly recommend googling one if you're not able to sit in front of a mirror right this second!)

Looking at your genitals can be scary for some, and I understand. The first time I looked at myself I was outraged at what I saw – all these folds of skin and thick curly pubes. It looked alien to me because I'd never seen a vulva before! If you're struggling too, you might like to check out something like the

Labia Library on the greatwallofvagina.co.uk– this piece of art is now an online resource of hundreds of vulvas. It proves that we all look totally different and that whatever our vulva looks like is normal.

We also all look beautiful. If my saying that makes you feel uncomfortable or you don't agree, that's okay, learning about your body is a process. In my opinion, learning to love and accept your own body is the path to experiencing more joy and pleasure from it. It's hard to let somebody else fully love you if you don't feel that way about yourself too. This can be so much easier said than done, but this book is the start! If it helps, whatever shape, size or colour a vulva takes, I like to think of it as a beautiful flower that blooms when it's turned on.

If you're unsure what I mean when I say vulva, this is because one of the biggest misconceptions is that the general area is the vagina. The vagina is actually just the inside canal – the outside area is our vulva and this includes (among other things) the clitoris, the clitoral hood, the outer labia and the inner labia, which are all important to masturbation. Get that mirror out and we can take a closer look.

The clitoris (glans clitoris, to be precise) is a nub at the very top of our vulva and it's usually covered by a hood of skin. This clitoral hood can vary in size, leaving the clitoris less or more exposed. The clit itself can also vary in size – it might be easy to spot or you might need to ferret around a bit to find it.

Based off research in other mammals, the clitoris is thought to have 10,000 sensitive nerve endings, compared to our friends with penises having only 4,000. I mean . . . let's just digest that for a second. That button you're looking at apparently has 10,000 nerve endings – WOW! No wonder we get so much pleasure when we touch this area. If you haven't already given your clitoris a stroke, why not do so now? Register what it feels like when you do. For some, it might not feel like very much unless you're turned on, but for me it feels like a small ball of energy has ignited – a warm and tickly sensation that feels good, even if I'm not mentally aroused.

Below the clitoris we have some flappier bits of skin which surround our vaginal opening – these bits of skin are the outer labia (the labia majora), the larger surface of skin that folds around the inner labia (the labia minora), which is the second layer of skin directly around our vaginal opening. Labia differ in size and shape just as the clit hood does – everyone's is so different! You can have quite long labia or really short labia, and some are straight and some curl like iris petals – all are unique and totally normal. Give them both a stroke, too. How does it feel for you? Perhaps it feels nice, but not as obvious a sensation as the one you get from touching your clitoris?

Now look back at your clit. This is what is most commonly referred to as the 'clitoris', but that's actually just the exposed bit – the clitoris as a whole is much bigger than that, with most of it behind our vulvas, running in line with the labia. Imagine that the clit you can see is the top of a wishbone, and that the two long sides of the bone are hidden, one behind either side of your labia. Trace this 'wishbone' now – from the clitoris at the top down one side and then the other.

This wishbone-clitoris is why we feel pleasure all over our vulva, so I would encourage you to include your labia when you masturbate – the sensation caused by the 'legs' of your clitoris is far less intense than its exposed head, but it can add to the experience. The inside bits, science seems to suggest, are also how some vulva owners can orgasm through penetration alone[5]. The vagina doesn't have many nerve endings of its own, but given that the clitoris in the fuller sense of the word surrounds the vagina, penetration can arouse it. It's also the reason why lots of us *don't* orgasm through penetration alone. Yes, the clitoris comes very close to the vagina, but close isn't the same as being inside it! If you've never had a so-called vaginal orgasm, I'm going to give you some tips in this book on how to give it a go, but if they don't work then don't lose any time wondering why not; the real wonder, given where the clitoris is compared to the vagina, is that 30 per cent of the people who own one can!

I think the most magical thing about the clitoris is that it swells and appears to bloom when we're aroused. Blood rushes to this part of the body, which includes erectile tissue, and it enlarges and the colouring becomes flushed. Sound familiar? Yep – it behaves in a similar way to a penis; vulva owners get boners too! That's because the penis is the male equivalent or male 'homologue' of the clitoris – human genitals all start out exactly the same within embryos, developing into either the clitoris or the penis depending on the hormones they're exposed to, and as such they have lots of things in common (the clitoral hood, for example, is the equivalent of a foreskin). The way sex is presented on screen and elsewhere would have you believe that reaching orgasm through the vagina is the equivalent of reaching orgasm through the penis, but I hope this clears up why the real equivalent is actually the clitoral orgasm. Which is why, to my mind, clitoris action doesn't just belong in masturbation and foreplay, it belongs during penetrative sex too, and it's also why masturbation can be so brilliant at equipping you with the tools you need to have great sex with a partner if or when you're doing that. If you know what makes your clit go wild, which I hope this book will help you with, then you can bring that into your external sex life.

Okay, now we know what's happening outside . . . what about inside? Open your legs wide (I'd suggest bending them to help with this). A few inches below your clitoris, between your little pee hole and your anus, will be a fleshy sort of hole that changes shape if you start tensing your downstairs muscles. That's the entrance to the vagina; inside is a soft and squishy canal that connects to the uterus by way of the cervix. Just as vulvas differ from person to person, so does your vagina: it can vary in length and shape and ultimately that can change where you feel pleasure. It's pretty hard to get a good picture of what is going on in there, because it's so out of sight. So wash your hands, we're going to explore . . .

You might have heard of the 'G-spot' inside the vagina – some biologists say that it's linked to the big clitoris (though not enough research has been done to prove this), with others disputing its existence. But let's not get stuck on that; many vulva owners (myself included) agree that there is a place inside your vagina that feels great when you rub against it. This place can change in location for different people, so there isn't a hard-and-fast rule on how to find it (and don't worry at all if you can't; as above, that's why some biologists don't believe it's real!). I recommend testing the waters and feeling for yourself. Use a clean finger or two (wet or lubed up if needed) to explore. If you place your fingers inside and feel upwards for a soft walnut-like thing on the front of your canal, that's usually the spot. The best way to describe the movement for finding it is to insert your fingers and move in a 'come hither' motion. It doesn't feel as sensitive as the clitoris, but it does feel more sensitive than its surroundings and that's what you want to stimulate to find 'G-spot pleasure'. Some sex toys are made to reach this exact place – if you want to know more see page 103.

If you want to carry on exploring, then up beyond the G-spot, you'll eventually find your cervix – it feels smooth and round. This is the entrance to your uterus. There are some interesting ways of stimulating your cervix which you can find on page 219.

I hope this has helped you to feel a bit more clued up on your anatomy, and that it's got you thinking about what to touch when you're masturbating and why it feels good. Feel free to keep looking at yourself! Perhaps read your first story in front of the mirror and see how much you bloom!

WHAT FANTASY ARE YOU FEELING TODAY?

To decide which masturbation meditation is right for you today, you might like to look back at the Contents page and choose simply based on the title, or look at the key at the top of each story to see roughly how long it will take to read, the personality of the sexual partner, or what sex each story contains. Alternatively, you can give the flow chart below a try.

START

Who would you like your POV character to be?

- **Ideally a woman** → Who would you like the partner(s) to be?
- **Ideally a man** → What sort of mood are you in?

Who would you like the partner(s) to be?
- **Both** → Threesome or moresome?
- **Woman** → Want a dildo to feature?
- **Man** → One man or two men?

Threesome or moresome?
- **Moresome** → When Good Neighbours Become Good Friends
- **Threesome** → Public or private?

Public or private?
- **Private** → My Boyfriend and Her
- **Public** → An Outside Orgasm for Three

Want a dildo to feature?
- **Yes** → Being Watched
- **No** →

One man or two men?
- **Two** → Between Two Cocks
- **One** → Up for some power play?

Up for some power play?
- **Not really** →
- **Maybe** → Who's in charge?

Who's in charge?
- **The woman** → Is a strap-on too far for you?
- **The man** → Do you want spanking?

Is a strap-on too far for you?
- **Show me the strap-on!** → Pegging
- **Too much for me** → The Sheriff and the Bandit

No, but up for literally ... → (Pegging / The Sheriff and the Bandit)

Do you want spanking?
- **Yes** →
- **Not bothered** → With the professor or the boss?

With the professor or the boss?
- **Boss** → Business Time
- **Professor** → Lust after Lectures

Are you after a proper 'dom'/'sub' fantasy?
- **Yes** →
- **No** →

What sort of mood are you in?
- **Romantic** → Afternoon Delight on the Beach
- **Naughty** → Do you like the sound of restraints?

Do you like the sound of restraints?
- **Yes!** → The Master
- **Not that naughty** →

20

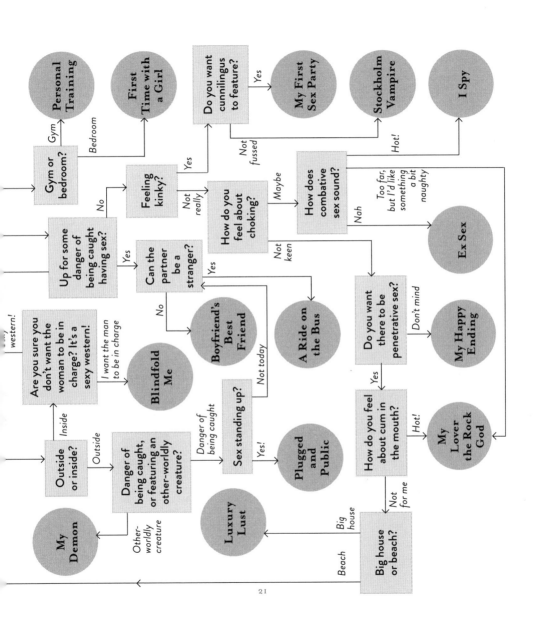

IT'S ALL IN YOUR HEAD

Here's a very important part of the equation: it's not just about physical touches and techniques when it comes to feeling pleasure. The most important tool you have is your MIND. Personally, I can be touching myself, or even having sex, and yet if my mind is elsewhere, I'll feel nothing. But if the mind can distract us from 10,000 nerve endings, think what it can do when we DO engage it. We need to be present for masturbation – albeit a pretty cool kind of present that can take us off to far-flung fantasies.

So how do we use our mind when we masturbate? Firstly, you need to figure out your turn ons and turn offs. I would suggest you start with your turn offs. Some people like masturbating when they're stressed or need to be somewhere – it can add a thrill to the occasion. For others, the biggest turn off is when we have something specific (like replying to an email or remembering to pick up loo roll) that won't stop flashing neon inside our brains, or we're worrying about something big and important. Please don't dismiss this. Don't think about your turn ons as if they can override the turn offs – lighting a nice candle doesn't mean you can now forget to pick up the loo roll. You need to get rid of your turn offs *and* include your turn ons for the best masturbation experience. So if you're stressed or worried about something and you find it's getting in the way of your pleasure, may I suggest you help yourself there first. For the small things, if I can't go and do them right away then I find writing a to-do list, so I don't have to keep the information in my head, helpful.

Other turn offs might be something to do with your surroundings – lots of mess? A sterile environment? Or smells – sewage? Washing powder you don't like? – things like that. Figure out what you don't like and change it up. FYI, this isn't just a tip for solo sex; it'll help you with your external sex life too!

Once you've made sure there are no turn offs around, you can settle into your turn ons. Firstly, think about what makes you feel good about yourself. It might be washing your hair or wearing perfume or clean pyjamas. It might be knowing you've done lots of exercise or having had an evening on the sofa with chocolate and ice cream. Tap into what makes you feel pleased with yourself. Also think about *where* does it for you. The bed might turn you on, sure, but so might the bathroom tiles or the kitchen table.

And then, of course, it's figuring out if there's a scenario or a certain fantasy that gets you going. Is it sex with an ex or being tied to the bed? There are no wrong or right answers here; your fantasies are going to be unique to you! There are certain things that get most of us off, and I've based the masturbation meditations on them for this book. They are here to inspire you and turn on your mind so that you can make the most of your pleasure mentally and physically. But there will be more besides that will feel unique to you; if you need a bit of help to figure them out then I've included a few pages at the back of this book to help you create your own sexual fantasies.

Sometimes we can feel ashamed or embarrassed about what turns us on. I don't think this is surprising when you consider that for thousands of years women were taught they could be either a Madonna (as in the virgin, not the pop legend) or a whore (in the patriarchy's mind, there was nothing worse) – there was no in-between when it came to sexuality. That sort of idea has really stuck around. You're either Sandy at the beginning of *Grease* – frigid and pure in her long dresses – or Sandy at the end of *Grease* – sexual and naughty in tight black leather. Sure, that's changing now, but it takes a long time to undo the millennia of history that have made women feel that being sexual is akin to being slutty → and being slutty is bad → but if you don't put out then you're boring → but being sexual is akin to being slutty, and so it goes round. On top of that, my education certainly didn't do anything to help any gender celebrate their naughtiest thoughts or explain that lots of people have deliciously dark desires.

So I'm here to say: you can be Sandy at the start of *Grease* AND Sandy at the end of *Grease* – or neither! How sexual you feel is as unique to you as your vulva is. More to the point, whatever turns you on is totally normal, even if you think it's outside of the 'norm'. And for the record, there is something very human about finding the opposite of what we want from real life erotica. It's why some big-shot male CEOs love to be dominated, and why some female feminists dismantling the patriarchy like to be tied up. Totally. Normal.

If you ever feel uneasy about what you're thinking about, I highly suggest tuning into our conversations on the F**ks Given podcast so that you can hear all of these things being normalised.

Right – turn offs banished and turn ons engaged? Start reading that story.

LUST AFTER LECTURES

READING TIME

<7 MINUTES

THE SEXUAL PARTNER IS

GOOD *AND* BAD

SEXY CHECKLIST

- ■ MASTURBATION
- ■ CLIT PLAY/FINGERING
- ☐ CUNNILINGUS
- ■ BLOW JOB
- ☐ NIPPLE PLAY
- ■ VAGINAL PENETRATION
- ☐ ANAL/BUTT PLAY
- ■ SPANKING
- ☐ SEX TOYS
- ☐ CHOKING
- ☐ BDSM

I look into the mirror in the university bathroom and pull my hair back tightly into a ponytail, feeling nervous but determined. I'm about to see my professor for my final, one-on-one assessment of the year and my heart is skipping with the anticipation of sitting opposite him alone in his office.

I've watched the way his muscles press against his shirt sleeve when he lifts his arm to the top corners of the board all year. The way the hair at the nape of his neck looks when it's damp from sweat after he's cycled to campus. The way he rubs his forefinger slowly against his thumb when he's listening to a question.

And it's not one-sided. He invites me to all his talks – he makes it sound purely professional, that I'll learn something from it if I go, but he doesn't suggest it to anybody else. He looks at me differently to all the other students, as if he's X-raying me, and he knows the way my eyes linger on him when he speaks isn't just respect, but something else. He often holds my gaze for longer than is acceptable, before he looks away, knowing it's not allowed.

The corridor is less busy than usual, some students already home for summer. My purposeful footsteps echo across the floor; some people turn to watch. I reach his door, his name printed with black text on the frosted-glass window obscuring the inside. My heartbeat is as loud as my knocks. I lean forwards to take the knob in my hand, and twist.

He smiles welcomingly, indicating the chair opposite him. I let my eyes roam over him as I move, wanting to memorise his face and body for the months ahead. My eyes glance to his shirt: it's unbuttoned one more than usual. Maybe it's because of the summer heat, maybe it's for my benefit. I want to slip my hand inside the crisp material and rub it over his chest.

I sit down and cross my legs. It means my skirt rides up a little higher. For the slightest of seconds I catch him glancing down at my exposed thigh. He's flustered as he sifts through the papers on his desk, searching for my assessments.

I ask him how he is, how his day is going. He tells me it's been long, but that I'm his final appointment. My pussy ignites. The perfect opportunity. It's now or never.

He takes me through my essays, compliments my work and my attitude. I tell him it's down to him, that I've loved his classes, have learned so much from him. He looks embarrassed but pleased and changes the subject: tells me where I've improved and what to think about for next year. 'Does that sound fair to you?' he asks me.

'I think, perhaps . . . ' I swallow. My heart feels very present in my chest. 'I think maybe I need to work on my focus in lectures.'

He looks directly at me. It shoots adrenalin down from my throat to my pants. 'Oh?'

'Sometimes,' I say, trying to hold my nerve, our eyes still attached to each other, 'sometimes I get distracted.'

I uncross my legs and cross them again. His gaze travels over the gap between. He tries to be quick about it, but he's not quick enough. The vibe in the room shifts, a tension has fallen over both of us. My pulse is quickening inside my pussy. I can see his mind racing against what's right and wrong.

And then he looks away. 'It's clearly not doing you any harm,' he says. 'You've had a brilliant year.' He starts talking animatedly about his summer plans as he stands up and tucks his laptop into a bag; I'm dismayed and confused, wishing he'd slow down.

'Sir . . . '

He hoists his bag over his shoulder and backs away from me towards the office door. 'Have a good summer. You can see yourself out?'

I look, open-mouthed, at the door that's closed behind him. I've scared him off! I think I could scream from frustration. My pussy burns longingly, wanting to be touched so badly. I look around at his cluttered office – at his notepads on the table, his pen pot, the books on the shelves – and then my eyes settle on a sweater over the back of the chair. If this is the closest I can get . . .

I stand up, wriggle my knickers down and step out of them. I go to his chair, pick up the sweater and breathe in his washing powder and aftershave. Excitement stirs within me, even more so now my pussy is bare. I sit down in his chair, spread my legs and touch myself with the hand that's not holding his sweater. My pussy is so wet and swollen from having been in his presence. Both pleasure and relief spread through me at my touch. I close my eyes and lean my head back.

The door opens. I look up. There's my professor. I don't know what to do; I sit there frozen. 'I forgot something . . . ' he tries to say but his voice trails off. He's staring at me, at my open legs, at my wanting, wet pussy.

He closes the door behind him. Does that mean . . . ?

Now he's turning the lock. I try to remember to breathe as he walks towards me slowly and stops just in front of me. My eyes are directly in line with his erection pressed against his tailored trousers. This is something I've fantasied about for the whole year: to find out what is underneath his freshly pressed clothing.

'Sir . . . ' I swallow, looking up at him. He gazes back down at me, his jaw rigid, a fierce lust in his eyes. 'Can I?'

He nods at me. I take his belt and slowly remove it, the leather rubbing against my skin with a satisfying coarseness, making my hairs stand on end. His clasps come away easily and his trousers fall to the ground. I take my hands around his boxers and pull them down. His cock springs to life as it's set free. He watches me taking it all in, it pulses in anticipation. I kiss it gently, teasing his head with my tongue before I take him into my mouth. I can feel him harden even more as I move on him. I look up at him as I suck, catching his eyes staring down at me. He takes his hand to my head and tightens his fingers around my ponytail, pulling me up to him. My mouth is wet, dripping with the taste of him.

He spins me around and pushes me down on to the desk, my naked ass arching up at him. A slap echoes over the room as his hand plants itself on my skin. I can feel the ghost of the sting and his eyes taking me in. He works his fingers over my wet pussy and up to my clit and I gasp at the contact of his hand on me for the first time. He plunges two fingers into me, electric shocks flicking through my body, radiating as he works himself inside. His other hand caresses my ass cheeks, teasing me before another slap echoes across the room. The pain shoots through me and heightens the pleasure from his fingers inside. I moan as he pushes deeper and slaps harder.

He pulls his fingers out and pushes his hard cock between my cheeks; it feels huge behind me. My hands clasp on the wooden desk as he plunges inside me. My head dizzies as he reaches down to my clit and starts working his hands in a circular motion at the same time.

'Fuck!' I exclaim as the dual stimulation edges me closer. He drives me into the desk as he thrusts, fucking and rubbing me harder and harder. My face is pressed down on the wooden surface among the papers, drool smudging ink, but all I can think about is the climax that's building inside me.

'Sir, I'm going to cum,' I breathe heavily as with one final deep plunge inside me, my pussy spasms around him. He moans as he feels me cumming. He takes his hand off my clit and pulls on my ponytail, quickening to bring himself to his climax. I feel him pulse inside me as he fills me, his cum warm inside, dripping down my leg.

He collapses on top of me, his weight heavy, the scent of his washing powder filling my nostrils. His breath tickles my neck as he kisses my skin softly. After a whole year I can't believe I finally got what I wanted. I've fucked my professor.

TIP 2:

TOUCH POINTS

Sometimes it can feel quite daunting just being with your own body, lying in bed with nothing but your own thoughts and fingers. BUT, getting over that hurdle and treating yourself as an exciting blank page instead is how you're going to get to know your body in ways you can't even imagine yet!

Touching yourself anywhere and everywhere in the name of research has another plus too. Have you ever been in a sexual situation with a partner and they've asked you what you like? You stare at them blankly and don't really know what to say? Me too; we've all been there. It's hard to know what you like in the bedroom when you haven't done the preliminary research. Knowing for sure how you feel pleasure by yourself is a massive step forward to being able to communicate what you like to partners. No more leaving it to them to figure it out for you!

Below are the places I would recommend giving a feel the next time you masturbate. I've given specific tips in this book on how to engage most of them and have included what page to flick to if you want to find out right away what they are. I would really recommend you do some gentle exploration of your own, though – going through as many of these areas as you feel comfortable with and noting the sensations that occur for you when you do. Each of us is unique in our preferences, so you'll learn just as much from yourself as from this book.

- Clitoris and labia. (Some people have very high sensitivity and might need to avoid direct contact with their clitoris – see page 76 for tips – while others can dive straight up on in there and stimulate away – see page 84 for these.)

- Vagina. (Internal play isn't for everybody but it can be amazing! See page 119 for ideas.)

- Anus. (Unlike penis owners we don't have a prostate, so we don't get as much pleasure from our anal passage as they do. That being said, it can still feel pleasurable for some vulva owners and really add to the overall experience. See page 157 for more.)

- Nipples. (Amazingly sensitive areas! See page 130.)

- Other body erogenous zones, while they aren't directly linked with sexual pleasure, still create amazing additional sensations during solo or partnered sex. These include:
  a. armpits
  b. inner thighs
  c. feet
  d. ears
  e. neck

Basically, our whole body can be used for pleasure depending on how you touch it! When it comes to feeling pleasure, the only thing you need is an open mind.

PERSONAL TRAINING

READING TIME
<7 MINUTES

THE SEXUAL PARTNER IS
UPBEAT AND POSITIVE

SEXY CHECKLIST
☐ MASTURBATION
■ CLIT PLAY/FINGERING
■ CUNNILINGUS
☐ BLOW JOB
■ NIPPLE PLAY
☐ VAGINAL PENETRATION
☐ ANAL/BUTT PLAY
☐ SPANKING
☐ SEX TOYS
☐ CHOKING
☐ BDSM

The only thing that can drag me out of bed at the weekend is my personal trainer. I've never been much of an exercise person but she has me coming back every week.

She meets me as I walk out of the changing room, telling me she's ready to work my ass till it drops. I look at her with doe eyes and say, 'Don't hurt me.'

'Oh, you know how I like it when you sulk,' she says with her white, gleaming smile. 'I'll only work you harder.'

She winks at me and walks us over to our first machine. We take on the treadmill for my warm-up; the sweat starts beading on my forehead and my cheeks feel hot. Elle stands next to me ramping up the speed; every time she makes it a little harder she gives me a wink. She talks to me about her day and what she's up to this evening, but I'm not listening. I'm looking at her lips as they move. They're so soft and moisturised, hypnotising me with every word. I see the pink flash of her tongue and my mind starts to wander. I feel my heart racing, thumping a little harder than usual . . . must be from the running.

We move over to the weights area; the usual suspects are grunting and checking themselves out in the mirrors. Mostly they're men flexing, probably more turned on by themselves than by anyone around them. I feel oblivious to their presence when I'm here; it's just me and her. She grabs some weights and starts demonstrating the lunges I'm going to be doing three sets of. Her eyes flicker to mine as she notices me accidentally staring straight at her perfect butt. I blush and grab the weights from her to get to work. She keeps her eyes on me the whole time, checking my form. The thrill of knowing she's

watching me sends heat into areas you wouldn't expect during
a workout.

After countless muscles are worked and sweat is moistening my
whole body, we end up on the mats for the final exercise of the day.
Abs and then stretches. My favourites – not because of the routine but
because I get to be so close to her.

'Girl, really great work today,' she says. 'This is the last push.'

It always makes my heart swell when she praises me, knowing that
she thinks I've done a good job.

She tells me to lie back on the mat as she stands above me, and then
to crunch and punch up to reach her hands. I feel my cheeks filling
with blood at this position we're in. Her towering above me, staring
down with her big smile, waiting for me to reach up to her. There
is something weirdly sexual about the power she has over me in this
moment. I'm sure she notices me staring longingly at her. At the way
her lips open slightly, her skin glistening and glowing. She smiles
broadly every time I make it up to touch her hands.

Once we're done, we both flop down on to the mat to stretch out
the forty-five-minute workout. She pulls me into some tense stretches,
her touch feeling magnetic all over my Lycra-ed body. We're suddenly
very still and extremely close. I can hear her breath low and slow, my
heart beating, pulse throbbing. We catch each other's eyes and linger
there, the heat from my skin radiating off me. Her eyes connect with
mine in a knowing look. We're both feeling something new. Her hand
is holding on to my thigh, pulling my leg in a stretch that's opening
up my hips. Her fingers suddenly feel like they're sending messages

into my skin. 'Do you want this?' And my eyes are saying 'yes', ready to be putty in her hands. She tentatively moves her hand slowly up my inner thigh as she stays connected to my eyes, questioning silently. All I want to do is grab her neck and pull her into a kiss. But we're in the gym, surrounded by grunting muscle men and ladies on the StairMasters.

'I'm going to go and shower,' I say, hoping she'll understand it's an invitation.

She gazes hard at me. 'I think I need to shower too,' she says, and then she pulls away. My stomach sinks that the moment is over, but then once she's standing, she reaches down to take my hand. A gesture to help me get up, but something so much more too.

I wait in the shower, nerves chasing up my spine. Did I misread things? Was it mad to think she'd join me? The water falls sharply over my shoulders, the heat pricking my sore muscles. I watch the water drip down my naked body, counting the seconds as they turn into breathless minutes.

Then the door opens behind me, and it closes just as quickly. I look down and see not only my feet but a pair of perfectly pedicured toes. Two hands move themselves around my stomach and my breath gets caught in my lips. Her hands start moving their way around my body, caressing ever so slowly over my lower back and stomach. Her mouth lingers on the back of my neck, breath tickling and sending sparks down into my body. Her hands are searching, moving over my breasts, stopping to tease my nipples. I bite my lip as she starts kissing my neck and shoulders.

My breath is long and slow, bringing the pleasure into myself deeper. One of her hands travels back down my stomach and further past my pubes into my folds, igniting small flames across my skin. She moves her fingers delicately over my clit and I let out a small moan of pleasure. Her other hand wraps around my mouth, quieting me. My pulse throbs in my pussy under her touch. Her fingers move around, and down, and suddenly two of them are slipping inside me and rhythmically pulsing against my tensing muscles, pleasure spreading within as she moves deeper. I moan into the hand that's still covering my mouth. She's playing with me with a skill I didn't expect; she knows exactly how to move her fingers around my clit and where to press deep inside me.

The shower splashes around us, soaking us and making her body slip against mine. It feels so warm and firm. It feels so right. My breath quickens.

I turn to her and she looks at me hungrily, her hands still attached to my body. I move in to finally kiss her. We lock into a deep embrace. My tongue meets her tongue and we are tangled in a hot mess of saliva and water. My hands move over her, feeling the slippery softness of her skin. My heart is racing, nervous, excited, and very fucking horny. I reach down to feel her pussy, brushing past her hair and finding her clit, and down into her soft warm depths. She's wet with anticipation for me.

She pushes me against the back wall of the cubical and kisses me hungrily, moving from my lips to my neck. Her hands work at my pussy, circling my clit and teasing my entrance. She moves down to my breasts, taking one nipple in her mouth and gently sucking. Then down to my belly, she kisses every inch of me and kneels in front of me.

'You're beautiful,' she says, looking at my pussy and then up at me. Before I can say anything my breath is stolen as she kisses my clit and starts caressing me with her tongue. It feels like there are a thousand fireworks going off in my pussy, pulsating through my whole body, from my toes to my fingertips. I pull her head into me deeper. Her hand works the inside of my thighs, pinching at my skin. Then she moves her fingers up deep inside me. I feel like my body could collapse on to the floor, my knees buckling in the pleasure, but she holds me up with her other hand. Pressing me back into the wall, supporting me.

My moans are stifled by biting my lip, trying to keep quiet so no one can hear us. No one can know what's happening in this shower cubicle.

She pushes further inside me with her hand, rhythmically teasing my G-spot, her mouth sucking on my clit. I'm in ecstasy. My breath quickens and I feel myself tensing and tightening around her. She keeps going as I reach my final breath and break into orgasm. **I gush around her as my muscles tense and spasm, letting myself go completely.** I feel her take one last big lick and remove her fingers.

She stands up and finds my lips with hers. Her breath is sweet on mine. We stand there panting as we intertwine our limbs in an embrace. All I can hear is our heavy breaths catching up with themselves, the water splashing on our skin and the tiles.

She pulls away from me and wipes her saliva off my lips. Then she winks. 'I'll see you next session.'

She slinks out of the cubicle and I stand there by myself smiling, the end of the fuse still tingling between my legs.

PLEASURE IS THE EVENT, ORGASM IS THE AFTERPARTY

While we're all here to feel and experience more pleasure I'm going to make a wild statement.

Orgasm is not the goal

Quite often we can find it really hard to experience orgasm or climax during any sexual play, no matter whether that's solo or with a partner. The main culprit for finding it hard to orgasm is our mind. And while you can banish your turn offs and bring in your turn ons (see page 22 for more on this), the pressure we can put ourselves under to reach climax can kill all of that. The best thing to do is to take the emphasis off it right from the get-go. An orgasm isn't an achievement – it's just an amazing addition to an already extremely great experience. If you emphasise the orgasm it takes attention away from the present pleasure that happens before it. There is as much pleasure on the journey to orgasm as there is to the actual orgasm itself! So let's take a step back and put our attention on the exploring, the building of pleasure, and if we orgasm at the end of our play that's amazing, but it's not everything. (The best part of this is that by taking the pressure away, you're so much more likely to be able to experience an orgasm as part of your solo sex.)

As you masturbate through the next story, why not completely abandon the idea of climax and just enjoy how you're feeling as you touch yourself instead?

NOTE: If you are finding it hard to experience any pleasure or orgasms please consult your doctor or a sex and relationships therapist. There can be a multitude of reasons for not experiencing one or both, including the effects of certain medications, or a past trauma. The most important thing is you recognise that you deserve pleasure, and it's best to get a professional opinion if nothing's working for you.

BOYFRIEND'S BEST FRIEND

READING TIME
<7 MINUTES

THE SEXUAL PARTNER IS
MYSTERIOUS

SEXY CHECKLIST
■ MASTURBATION
■ CLIT PLAY/FINGERING
□ CUNNILINGUS
■ BLOW JOB
□ NIPPLE PLAY
■ VAGINAL PENETRATION
□ ANAL/BUTT PLAY
□ SPANKING
□ SEX TOYS
□ CHOKING
□ BDSM

I roll over and feel the sun graze my back, the smell of suncream and chlorine tingling in my nose. I catch his eye again as I move, seeing his gaze trace over my body in my tangerine bikini. On my other side, my boyfriend sleeps softly with a book resting on his face. I can see he's getting burnt in the heat of the Italian sun. I sit up to locate the cream for him, appreciating the view from our villa as I do so. We're in the middle of rolling verdant hills, with grapevines and neat, tall Cypress trees weaving through the distance. The rest of our friends are scattered around the edge of the pool, sipping on the local wine and laughing with each other.

I gently place the suncream bottle in my boyfriend's hand. When he stirs, I point at his reddening skin. He rolls his eyes at me, hating to be mothered, but squirts the liquid over himself, massaging it in. My eyes linger on his chest, the sprouts of hair mingling with the cream.

As I lie back down, I cast an eye over to see if David, my boyfriend's best friend, is still looking. I've noticed him doing it all holiday. But no, right now he's lying on his stomach in the shade, his face turned the other way. I know it's bad, but I'm disappointed. His attention makes me feel good. My eyes travel over his hair, wet from the pool, to the curve of his back and down to his butt. I've never really looked at it before. It's pert, hidden inside dark blue swim shorts that I know would be silky if I ran my hand over them . . .

I close my eyes quickly to stop myself looking. That only makes the daydreaming worse.

A beautiful evening sunset floods the skies as everyone filters out to the courtyard where a dining table has been set up with candles of all different heights and sizes; twinkling fairy lights hang in the vines that trace up the arches of the stone walls of the house that encases us. It's one of the most romantic settings I've ever seen. Beaming, I look at my boyfriend – he's pulling out his chair, oblivious and unappreciative of the effort our hosts have gone to. I say his name, hoping that if he looks up and sees me – dressed to impress, my skin dewy and supple from moisturiser, perfume glistening on my neck and wrists – he might come into the moment with me. But he doesn't hear me, or – worse – chooses to ignore me. My heart sinks as he takes a seat down the table from me, starting a conversation with another of our friends. Someone brushes past me, the fabric of a linen shirt tickling my skin. I look up: it's David. He pulls out the chair next to me. Before sitting down, he stands over me and takes me in, including my glazed eyes from the small moment of pain my boyfriend's just caused me.

'You look beautiful,' he says. His words seem to plunge into my mouth, down my throat and bang into my pussy, drumming on it. I cross my legs, trying to make the feeling go away.

All through dinner, David's presence next to me feels heavy, obvious. I notice each stir of his arm, the small movements of his leg under the table. Every now and then, out of duty, I look over at my boyfriend; he's sweating under his shirt, the pink of his chest radiating from his collar. He looks uncomfortable.

After dessert, a few of our friends filter off to bed, leaving the table emptier and emptier. My boyfriend, for the first time this evening, comes over to me and tells me he's heading to bed. 'Are you coming?' he says.

Just as I open my mouth to reply, I feel David's hand on my thigh. It sends a sharp jolt into my skin and up my leg. I look down at my empty plate, my heart beating hard in my chest. What is happening? Why do I want to find out?

'I think I'll stay down a little longer, have one more glass,' I hear myself saying. My boyfriend pats my shoulder, waves at David and goes.

'Goodnight then,' a voice next to me says. I turn. David's pushing his chair back from the table. What? He's leaving?

'You're . . . you're going?' I say. Later, I wonder if he used this moment as a test for us both, to find out what I wanted.

'Yes,' he says. 'Goodnight.'

'All right then,' I say tersely. 'Bye.' I look away from him, lean my elbows heavily, almost tantrum-like, on the candlelit table.

'I want to fuck you senseless.'

I whip my head around. He's already moving away. Did he just say that? Did I imagine it?

I go to bed but I can't sleep. I know what I want now. I want to stand behind David's butt and put it in my mouth like an apple. The guilt of it makes me feel dirty. But feeling dirty also feels exciting.

I get out of bed and go downstairs on to the veranda with the pool that looks out over the hills. There's a bright silver moon in the sky and I lie down on one of the loungers, pull down my pyjama shorts and put a finger to the opening of my pussy. It's so glad to be touched; it's been aching all day. The opening of it is wet already, and I slide that wetness up to my clit. I keep doing this, teasing myself, with my eyes closed, until . . .

I feel somebody's breath on my lips. I open my eyes. It's him. He's on the lounger, his face an inch from mine. Adrenalin floods through me. We look at each other, waiting to see if one of us is going to stop this, but instead giving each other permission. And then he leans forward and touches his lips to mine. I kiss him back, grab the back of his neck and slip my tongue into his wet mouth.

He moves his hand down my pyjama top and flutters it over the bottom of my naked stomach, the tickles creating sparks in my pussy. Then he moves his hand down and slips his finger inside. I moan. He puts his other hand over my mouth. His finger rubs playfully around my G-spot, exploratively rather than rhythmically, as if what he's most interested in is what I feel like. I keep my body relaxed, not trying to find a climax, so I can make the most of the feeling of him rubbing me for as long as possible. I open my mouth and lick his hand; he gives me his thumb to suck on and I love how filled up I am in this moment.

'Stand up,' I say.

He likes that I'm telling him what to do. He stands next to me where I'm sitting on the lounger, facing me. I pull his shorts down hungrily and they fall to the floor. His penis springs out, saluting me, but first I want his ass. I put my hands on his hips and turn him around. Still sitting on the lounger, I run my hands over the curves of his cheeks. I grab them in my hands. I run my tongue over them and gently bite the skin there. I can't believe my wish has come true.

I turn him back around. I wrap my wet tongue around his cock. I hold his butt cheeks and pull him towards me so that I have the whole length of him inside my mouth. Like the way he was touching me, I don't do it rhythmically, I do it mindfully. I notice how it feels for me, how powerful I feel, how successful I feel to be able to take the whole of him in my mouth, how wet my tongue is, how smooth the skin of his cock is, how it's slightly salty, how he reacts when I suck on the tip and when I run my tongue side to side and up and down.

He's running his hands through my hair and down my neck, swaying with the pleasure of it. With a little moan he takes his dick out of my mouth and waits for me to say what's coming next. I stand up and tell him to lie down. I get on top of him but with my back to him. I take his cock in my hand, roll it over the entrance of my pussy to wet it and sit down. The first plunge is like an explosion for us both. The angle of his cock on my G-spot as I begin to move is so intense I feel like I'm floating. His hands are running over my butt, squeezing my cheeks, up and down my back, nipping at my waist as if he can't believe I'm real. I touch his thighs beneath me doing the same thing and then I move two fingers to my clit as I rock, slow and steady and then faster and faster on his hard cock. I'm so wet, I rub myself with more passion and life than I've ever done before, tensing my pussy muscles around him as I ride and ride him. **I'm engulfed in pleasure as I cum, my legs trembling. I open my eyes and look up at the shining moon and the hills it's illuminating.**

Afterwards, I lie on the lounger, waiting for my breath to go back to normal, keeping my fingers pressed lightly against my pulsing clit. I would think I'd imagined it, imagined his fingers inside me, his cock in my mouth – but I could never make up how good it felt to have his ass cheek in my mouth.

TIP 4:

SEDUCE YOURSELF

I don't know about you but before having sex with a partner I want one of us to set the scene. Turn the lights down, maybe light a candle, and most definitely put some great sexy music on. Why don't we do this for ourselves when we're diving into a solo sex session? For this upcoming meditation, let's all take a moment to set our scene. Where do you want to be? Where is your ultimate relaxation spot – or maybe somewhere that feels new and exciting? What lighting makes you feel sexy? What smells get you going? If you want to listen to some music, my favourite albums for sexy times are: Moonchild: *Voyager*, Khruangbin: *Hasta El Cielo* and Gary Clark Jr: *The Story of Sonny Boy Slim*. What are yours? Make your scene your ultimate sexy space for yourself, not just for partners.

The other thing we do if we're having sex with someone else is set aside time for it. Yeah, we might have a quickie from time to time, but it's often an actual plan where other events aren't allowed to interrupt it. Let's do that for ourselves, too! I'd strongly advise at some point setting an hour aside to spend time with yourself. No distractions, just you and your body.

AFTERNOON DELIGHT ON THE BEACH

READING TIME
<7 MINUTES

THE POV CHARACTER IS
LOVING & MALE

SEXY CHECKLIST
- ■ MASTURBATION
- ■ CLIT PLAY/FINGERING
- □ CUNNILINGUS
- ■ BLOW JOB
- □ NIPPLE PLAY
- ■ VAGINAL PENETRATION
- □ ANAL/BUTT PLAY
- □ SPANKING
- □ SEX TOYS
- □ CHOKING
- □ BDSM

My eyes twitch as the afternoon sun laps through the palm trees towering above us. I stir and roll on to my side. Next to me, my girlfriend is still sound asleep. My muscles are tight in my lap as my erection presses against my swim shorts. My girlfriend always teases me about my morning wood, but who wouldn't wake up like that when you're sleeping next to a goddess? Seems morning wood can happen in the afternoons too . . .

I look down to the sea, at the waves rolling gently against the shore. The sound of it is mesmerising. My girlfriend stirs, stretching her body out on the big blanket we've laid upon the sand. Her breasts slip out from under the triangles of her bikini and my eyes can't help but linger on them. As her eyes bat open I lean down and plant a kiss on her lips.

'Mmmmmm. Afternoon, beautiful,' I say, pressing my nose into hers. Every time I wake up next to her, even when it's just a nap, I feel like the luckiest guy in the world. She kisses me back, running her hand over my face as she smiles. She sits up and leans over me to reach into our bag, pulling out a bottle of water. Her ass is up in the air and her back arches as she moves. My cock twitches as I watch her, I can't help myself. I brush my hands over her soft skin, starting with her juicy ass, covered only by her bikini. I kiss it gently. She giggles at how quickly I took the bait. I knew she had leaned over like that on purpose.

My hands trace over her stomach and then reach into her bikini top and cup her breasts. They fall heavily in my hands, the skin so delicate and supple. I massage them slowly, teasing her nipples.

My touch makes her squirm in enjoyment, her pleasure turning me on more. She moves her shoulders down to lean on the blanket, keeping her ass up in the air and wiggling it a little to get my attention elsewhere. I look around to see if anyone's on the beach, but it's just us here in paradise.

I pull her bikini bottoms to one side, then I sit back and gaze at her beautiful pussy. The folds of her vulva sit squished together, presenting her wetness in-between. She looks ready for me and that's what drives me wild. She reaches down and undoes the bow on one side of her bikini bottoms, and then the other. The material floats down to the blanket.

I grab her thighs and pull her abruptly back so my mouth is inches away from her glistening pussy. My favourite view. My cock twitches again with desire, my eyes lap her up. I blow gently on her, which makes her squirm.

She begs me to kiss it. How can I say no? I plunge my tongue over her, licking from her clit up to her ass. I moan into her as her taste covers my tongue. I lap at her lips and then suck her clit softly. Her hands grab the blanket beneath her, pulling the fabric into her fists, until she finds the sand and pools it between her fingers. I love seeing her in pleasure, it drives me to go harder. I tease my tongue in her entrance, plunging in to taste her more.

'Fuck, you taste so good,' I tell her.

'That *feels* so good,' she replies, elongating the words.

I love having my face buried in her ass, her plump cheeks around my own. I lick around her clit in a circular motion, which increases her moans. Slowly seducing her pussy, kissing it like I would her other lips.

'I want you,' she breathes heavily back to me.

She manoeuvres herself around so she's facing me, taking off her bikini top at the same time. I stand and take off my swim shorts then sit back down, my hard cock standing up in admiration of her. She leans down between my legs, keeping her eyes on mine. I let out a muffled moan in anticipation of her touch, feeling the pulse in my cock as it throbs for her. She takes me in her hand, sending shivers of pleasure into my body. I love seeing her with my cock so close to her mouth. First she starts by dribbling on to me, working her hand up and down. She gets me wet and slippy, her grip tightening around my shaft. My cock aches in longing, a heat growing inside me getting me harder and harder. She teases the head with her tongue, my anticipation edging as all I want is her to take it fully into her mouth, but she knows the tease turns me on like crazy. I move my hand down to her face and push her hair back so I can see her properly.

'Take it all in, baby,' I say.

She's always so good at following orders. She takes my cock into her mouth, moving her tongue over my head. My eyes roll back as it sends sparks soaring down my shaft. Fuck. Yes. I look back and see her moving up and down, moaning on to me. The vibrations tingle among the warm wetness of her mouth. Her tongue moves around me, each time it rubs past my head it makes me swell and harden in her mouth. I could be in this moment all day, her lips around me, in her control.

She kisses the tip of my cock.

'I need you inside me,' she says a little breathlessly.

I want to be inside her badly. She sits up and leans over me, kissing my lips with her beautiful cock-covered mouth. I hold her body into mine so that she's sitting on me, meshing our skin together, melting into her softness. I kiss over her face, and down her neck, teasing her ears with my tongue. I feel her skin prickle at the sensations. I growl against her. I need all of her. My erection is pressing between her legs; I can feel the wetness dripping down my shaft and on to my balls.

I lie back while she stays sitting. She holds me between the folds of her pussy, rocking her hips on my shaft. I can feel the blood pumping to my hardness, the desire to pull her right on almost uncontrollable.

'I want it inside you,' I say. 'Now.'

She looks at me with a grin and hovers over me, the head resting at her entrance. I can feel pre-cum dripping out, tingling in the head of my cock. Her lips are open, her tongue resting at the bottom of her mouth. Finally, she slides on to me, pulling me completely inside her. We gasp in unison at the sensations; she feels so tight around me, so warm. She sits down with all her weight to take me fully into her, deep as she can. I gaze at this beautiful woman sitting on my lap, her thighs straddling me, her pussy clamped around me, her hips perfect for grabbing. Her breasts are directly in my eyeline bouncing at each movement. I can't help but move forward and take her nipples into my mouth, tasting the sweat that has beaded on her skin and the salty seawater from earlier in the day. The saltiness tastes good on my tongue. She rocks on me, keeping me deep inside her. My cock is grabbed and pulled by her, the sensations radiating throughout my whole body. She's so wet.

'You feel so, so good,' I tell her. She looks back at me and bites her lip.

'I know.' Her confidence drives me wild. She knows the power she has over me, the feelings she gives me. I grab her hips and pull her back and forth on me, groaning as my body is engulfed in pleasure. My breath is heavy as my chest sweats under her hands. I move my hips up to meet hers, pulling myself out and plunging back in. I can see the excitement growing in her eyes, her skin flushing on her chest. I want to watch her cum on me, I want to feel her restrict around me.

I reach for her clit, using the wetness from my dick going in and out of her. I massage the skin around. Circling around her clit, teasing it indirectly. She groans deeper and harder with an eagerness and tightens around me. Each time she tightens I feel a shock of heat ride through my body.

I move my hand faster, using more fingers to apply more pressure. She looks ethereal, riding on me, grinding her hips on me. The hotness is spreading down my shaft and spreading through me. She clenches and tightens on me, throwing her head back and letting out a deep moan. Her pussy is pulsing on me, taking me right to the edge. She pulls me in deeper.

'Cum for me.' Her gaze locks on mine with such passion and love. I lose control of myself, my head swirling as if I am close to passing out, ready to explode. **My cock tenses, I release and project into her, filling her up. I can feel my cum warm, deep inside her against my**

cock. My dick is tingling with the aftershock. She collapses down on to me, keeping me inside her, our sweaty bodies wet and warm. Feeling her heaviness on me feels comforting as we melt into one.

We slide off each other and lie facing the dazzling blue sky. I have that warm feeling of love filling my chest as I regain my normal breathing.

'I love you a lot, you know,' I say, turning to look at her.

'I know.' She smiles. 'I love you, too.' She stands up and begins to run to the sea. 'Race me?' she says.

How did I get so lucky?

TIP 5:

BREATHE

You need to be in a relaxed state of mind to feel pleasure and one of the easiest ways to get out of your head and into your body is by connecting to your breath. Unfortunately, porn has shown us plenty of wrong ways to breathe during masturbation and sex: all those short sharp breaths, or cutting off your air supply entirely by holding the breath. (I'm not including choking here – that can be hot!)

I'm definitely guilty of breathing this way too, but the best way to move into a parasympathetic nervous state (basically a prime relaxation state), which is essential to feeling comfortable and the max amount of pleasure, is actually to begin with lengthening your exhales. If we try to breathe slower and deeper, the pleasure becomes deeper and more intense too. I find if I'm ever struggling to feel pleasure during masturbation or sex, if I focus on my breath I can reconnect with the sensations.

Give the following simple technique a read now so you know what to expect, and then see if you can bring it into your solo sex when you get to the meditation – it's probably the most mindful and meditative practice you can do when it comes to self-pleasure. Getting out of your head and into your body is incredibly valuable!

STEP 1: Deepen your breath by breathing in through your nose for five to six seconds, and then out through your mouth for the same amount of time. Do this a few times so you're in a rhythm with it.

STEP 2: Keep breathing this way, and now visualise your breath starting from your genitals rising all the way up your body.

STEP 3: Think of the breath being the pleasure you're feeling, continuously breathing it up from your genitals into your head and all the way back down.

Naturally your breath will change when and if you start incorporating stimulation in different ways, but always try to connect back to the breath if you feel yourself getting back into your mind and out of your body.

In my research for this book, I spoke to my good friend Jamie Clements, a breathwork teacher, to find what breathing techniques he recommends for creating ultimate relaxation and pleasure. He reiterated that most people have the temptation to hold their breath, or breathe shallow or short during sex and masturbation – but what we actually want to be doing is breathing deeply and gently to keep ourselves in the state of relaxation. The technique he taught me is similar to the one above but with a different focus. It's called Microcosmic Orbit (I love the name – feels orgasmic):

STEP 1: Bring your attention to your pelvic floor muscles or your navel.

STEP 2: As you inhale deeply, visualise your attention and breath moving through your genitals and up your spine to your head.

STEP 3: As you exhale deeply, visualise the breath moving down the front of your body and back to your pelvic floor.

STEP 4: Repeat to create a flow of energy moving around your body.

NOTE: Make sure you're being safe with both these techniques: if you feel too light-headed slow it down and get back to your normal breathing rhythm.

A RIDE ON THE BUS

READING TIME

>10 MINUTES

THE SEXUAL PARTNER IS

FORWARD

SEXY CHECKLIST

☐ MASTURBATION
■ CLIT PLAY/FINGERING
☐ CUNNILINGUS
☐ BLOW JOB
☐ NIPPLE PLAY
■ VAGINAL PENETRATION
☐ ANAL/BUTT PLAY
☐ SPANKING
☐ SEX TOYS
☐ CHOKING
☐ BDSM

I take the same bus home every weekday. Up until a month ago, I would look at my phone for the whole journey, not noticing the rain sprinkling against the window or the changing leaves of the trees in the parks we were driving past. But then one day, my phone broke, and I looked up.

Two stops after mine, a guy about my age boarded the bus. I noticed him at first only because he has the same rucksack as me, but since then I've noticed other things. The way he looks out of the window for the whole journey, sometimes with his forehead pressed against the glass. The fact he doesn't have a preferred seat, unlike me (I always take the one a row from the back, to the right of the aisle as you face forwards). I don't *always* look at him, and when I do, it's not on purpose. If I notice the way his hair falls against his neck, and what his hands look like when they press the button, it's just an accident. When he gets off the bus, one stop before mine, and I daydream about what those hands would feel like on me, that's an accident too.

Today, I sit down in my regular seat, and I wait. Two stops later, I breathe a sigh of relief as he gets on. He's wearing a light jacket over a dark green jumper and he sits a few rows in front of me to the left, which gives me a good view of his neck. *I'm such a creep*, I scold myself, forcing myself to look away. But a few moments later, my eyes drift back.

He's sitting next to a guy in a suit and anorak and at the next stop, the anorak's friend gets on. The two men start talking and my guy gives up his seat so the friend can take it. He looks to the front of the bus, deciding which seat to choose. It's not a very full bus; there are plenty of options for him to take an empty row, if he'd like to.

Then he turns around, looking to the back of the bus, looking at . . . me. For the first time ever, our gazes cross paths. My pulse does a drum roll. Slowly, as the bus moves down the road, he walks towards me, not taking his eyes off me the whole time. When he gets to my seat, he smiles. He asks if I mind him sitting down.

'Sure,' I croak. I clear my throat. 'I mean, it's a free country.' I feel oddly embarrassed at what I've said and how I've said it as I pick up my bag to make room for him.

He sits down and his arm grazes mine. The sensation it causes is so obvious to me that I have to shuffle away. I get my new phone out and text a friend something unnecessary about weekend plans. Then the bus lurches and my phone slips out of my hand and on to the floor, by his foot. He reaches down to get it.

I hold my hand out and say thank you. But instead of putting it in my hand, he presses the phone into my lap, directly against my pussy. I'm wearing a jumper dress with no tights. Even through the woolly material and my knickers, the cold of the plastic seeps through and wakes my clitoris up. My mouth opens and my stomach somersaults. He looks directly at me and gives me another small smile, then lets the phone drop. Did he do that on purpose? Did he mean to be so suggestive? I swallow and pick up my phone. The absence of the coldness on my clit feels just as visceral as when it was there.

I lean down to where my bag is and put the phone away in the front pocket. That's also where I keep my keys. My mind is whirring. If he *was* being suggestive, then there's a way to find out for sure. I take the keys out and slide them across the floor in front of his feet, out of my reach.

I sit back up. 'Excuse me,' I say. He looks at me with an unreadable expression on his face. Somehow, heart pumping, I pluck up the courage to ask, 'Would you mind passing me my keys?'

He looks down at where they lie, spread around my palm-tree keyring. He seems to be thinking. Then he leans down and picks them up. I try to keep my breath smooth and even as I wait to see what he does next. I want him to do exactly what he did before: to press the keys into my lap. But instead he leans across to my leg. He takes one of the keys between his left thumb and forefinger, as if he's about to insert it into a lock, and then he starts to run it up my calf.

I tremble – whether from the cold, tickling sensation of it or from the surprise, I don't know. As he reaches my knee he gets to the hem of my dress. He hesitates, waiting long enough for me to stop him. I don't.

He continues to run the key across my skin, over the inside of my thigh. When he gets to my knickers, he presses the flat side into my pussy, so that my clit and my lips feel the cold, hardness of the metal.

I look around me to see if any of the people in front of us have noticed. The fact that they're here has kept me from gasping in response to his touch – otherwise I might have moaned.

He's looking at me. I meet his eyes with mine. He hasn't removed the key from my pussy, but now he lets it drop on to the material of my dress that's resting on the seat. He doesn't remove his hand, though. Instead, his eyes still looking into mine, he traces the inside of my thigh with his fingertips, moves them over my pants, where my pussy is now throbbing, and on to the other thigh. When he comes back to my pussy, this time he stops and begins to rub my clit through my pants.

I concentrate on my breathing. I hope it will stop me from making noise, but actually it's just deepening the pleasure.

His eyes leave mine to look down at his own crotch. I follow his gaze. I can see that his cock is starting to strain against the material of his trousers. This knowledge, coupled with his hand on my clit, makes me pant. I look up sharply at the passengers again to check no one heard me. The bus is stopping. I watch as the remaining passengers, except for the anorak and his friend, stand up to get off. Between my legs, his fingers pull my knickers to one side and plunge into my wet pussy.

I bite my lip to stop myself from making any noise. The pain mixes with the pleasure. He pulls his fingers out of me and moves up to my clitoris, where he travels around it in slow, wet circles. I grip the bar of the seat in front of me, then think it'll look too obvious if the two guys ahead look back at us. Instead, I lean back against the seat and continue to breathe in the pleasure radiating through my body from my pussy, and back out again.

Loudly, as if for the benefit of other people, he suddenly says, 'Excuse me, would you mind if we swapped places? I'd like to look out of the window.'

I frown at him. I'm confused as to why he's asked this as he'll have to remove his hand from inside my pants. Now he's frustrated me and given himself an erection, is it all over? But I can hardly say no. I nod, waiting for him to stand up to let me out, but he doesn't. So I get up first and he makes to shuffle over on the seat, and as he does so I see his plan: with his hands free he can now undo his trousers.

As I step to the left, the keys that were still inside my dress where he left them fall; they hit the floor with a loud clatter. The anorak and his friend look over at us and I freeze, wondering if from this angle they can see what I can now see: a hard, wanting, naked cock. But they look away; clearly his groin is hidden by the seats in front.

I sit down next to him, wondering what's going to happen next. He takes my hand and guides it down to my own pussy, where my knickers are still pushed to one side. He pushes my finger inside myself and circles it around, collecting my wetness. Then he pulls my finger out and guides my hand over to his cock. It feels hard but velvety. I wipe my wetness on to his shaft, and then wrap my palm and fingers around it and start to move my hand up and down. I look at his face, expecting to see an expression of pleasure – but he smiles with such politeness at me. Nothing else on his face would give away what we're doing.

The bus stops again and this time the anorak and his friend get off. For a heart-stopping second I think the anorak has spotted what we're doing now he's standing up – but then he picks up his bag and disappears down the stairs.

We're now alone. I know what I want to happen next. He looks around the empty bus and says, completely seriously, 'There's not very much space. You should probably sit on my lap to make room.'

I gulp, my hand still on his cock. Am I really going to do this? Have sex on the bus? My pussy flutters in answer. I give him one short nod and stand up. He pulls my dress up to my hips as I do and opens his legs. I step into the gap between them. Then he guides me gently down until he's filled me up. This time I do let out a moan – just the one – before I pull it together and concentrate on my breathing: there are still people who could hear us downstairs. The pleasure is surmountable so long as I concentrate. But then two of his fingers find their way to my clit and start to rub. He draws the wetness from my pussy and starts to circle it, round and round.

My climax begins to build; the position we're in means my pussy is creating the tightest of sleeves around his cock. I know he's getting close, too; I can feel his breath on my neck getting harder, feel his tensing muscles as he helps me to rock up and down on his hard shaft. The bus stops and people get on. I see the back of a head appear on the stairs, climbing up to the top deck. As his body appears, I see from his uniform that he's a police officer! But for us to stop now would be tantamount to torture. I keep moving on his cock in rhythm with him, and he keeps moving his finger over and around my wet clit. The officer who's come up the stairs doesn't look over – he sits down at the front of the bus and looks at his phone. His presence makes everything even wilder. **I keep my eyes on the officer as I feel the slippery, sweet sensation on my clit, feel the cock belonging to the stranger beneath me rubbing fiercely inside my pussy, feel his harsh breath on the back of my neck, feel my muscles beginning** to spasm, feel the pleasure beginning to erupt through my body – and I finally explode.

As the tiniest of moans escapes my lips, the officer at the front of the bus looks over at us, and I feel the cock inside me tense and lurch: he's cumming now too. The officer continues to look at me. I close my mouth and take a deep breath, knowing I can't get up until he leaves as I'll risk showing him my bare pussy.

Clearly the stranger I'm sitting on understands this too. Slightly out of breath, he leans up and kisses my cheek and says loudly and completely seriously, 'What shall we pick up for dinner?'

As I try to think of an answer, I feel a dribble of his cum drip down my pussy and on to the bus seat.

TIP 6:

THE WETTER THE BETTER

Lube can be a 'sticky' topic to broach, both for partnered sex and masturbation – yet in fact it's a game-changing pleasure enhancer for ALL sexual play. Plus, using lube can avoid microtears in your vagina which sometimes lead to thrush and bacterial vaginosis. Wetter is always better, even for your health!

I completely understand the hesitation when it comes to using lube. When I was a teenager, I had a partner who brought out the lube during our play and I was outraged, completely offended. I thought to myself, how dare he suggest I'm not wet enough; surely it's only grannies that need to use lube.

This isn't surprising considering we were never taught that lube is for everybody, expecting ourselves to be wet all the time whenever we wanted. That's not the case. During our cycle it's totally normal to have wetter parts and dryer parts, and also to get wet when we're not even in the mood; it's just the way our bodies work. I've learned the hard way that I don't always get wet when I want to have sex (if the same is true of you that is 100 per cent normal) and yet it could have been as easy as squirting out some lube, instead of thumbing a dry toy or penis into my vagina. So I firmly encourage you if you don't have some already to quickly pop to your local shop and buy some before you start on the next story! Using lube during masturbation can be revolutionary. It's so amazing for self-massage and getting sensual with your genitals, and especially so if you're using toys because they slip right up and in or around on the skin.

There are so many different types of lube to experiment with as well – it can be a really exciting part of masturbation. The main types are water-based, silicone-based and oil-based. If you're using your hands, you can try any of them. Glass, metal or crystal toys can also be used in conjunction with any lube – but if you're using silicone toys you'll want to use water-based because other lubes could corrode the material and become unusable. PS: if you're using condoms you want to make sure you're using a water-based or silicon-based option so the condom stays intact.

Under those three umbrellas, there is literally a whole world of lube out there – so many exciting products to try. What you want to look out for are natural ingredients that are pH-friendly so that you keep your vagina happy! There are lubes that do special things, like tingle, get hot or taste good. There are lubes specifically for anal or oral sex. The consistency you want to look out for is slippy not sticky. I personally love using CBD lubes as they feel super relaxing and in my experience can heighten sensations.

BUSINESS TIME

READING TIME

<10 MINUTES

THE SEXUAL PARTNER IS

ARROGANT

SEXY CHECKLIST

■ MASTURBATION
□ CLIT PLAY/FINGERING
□ CUNNILINGUS
■ BLOW JOB
□ NIPPLE PLAY
■ VAGINAL PENETRATION
□ ANAL/BUTT PLAY
■ SPANKING
□ SEX TOYS
□ CHOKING
□ BDSM

It's Friday; the skyrise office I work in is filled with light-hearted chatter as the clock gets closer and closer to 5.30 p.m. I've been working with my boss all week on a presentation for Monday and I can't wait for it to be over so I can get out of here. One more tweak and I'll send it to print.

My boss is pacing in his glass-walled office, impatiently waiting for me to give him the presentation so he can give it one more proofread before he leaves. He pulls a hand through his short, well-kept hair, revealing a small sweat patch on his shirt underarm. He's an arrogant sort of guy – smart and good looking, but he knows it – and yet I like the fact that he's human enough to sweat through his work clothes. He always smells so good when he leans down over my desk to talk to me. At that moment, he looks up and catches me staring at him. I turn back to my screen quickly, feeling my cheeks burn.

Final change made, I click PRINT on the document, tap my pen on the side of the desk and swivel in my chair, waiting. A spinny icon of doom appears. Hmm. I touch the mouse to see if I can prompt any movement. The screen goes completely blank. Fuck. I click the on button frantically, looking over my shoulder to check whether my boss has seen. I almost jump out of my skin: he's right behind me.

He asks me where the printout is. 'I just pressed print – but then this happened,' I grimace.

He leans over my shoulder – there's the salty smell of him I like, tickling my nose. He moves the mouse and clicks a few buttons. Nothing happens. He asks me if I emailed it to anyone, or saved it on the Cloud.

'It was on my desktop . . . ' My voice trails off into nothing.

His body stiffens with anger. My own shoulders tense, waiting for him to shout at me.

Instead, ever so quietly, he says, 'Be here tomorrow. Nine a.m. sharp.'

I'm here on time but he's beaten me to it: he's already in the kitchen making a coffee. He's stirring the spoon in the cup vigorously, obviously still angry. He doesn't look up at me when I walk past to get to my desk. I drop my stuff on my chair. My computer won't switch on. The office is dead, not a soul around, just us two in this silent, glass tower.

'Come with me.' His voice sends shockwaves through the cavernous maze of desks. Startled, I follow him into his spacious office where the whole of the outer wall is windows, looking out over a city of skyscrapers and bustling roads. He leads me to his desk, which I take as a command to sit down. The hairs prickle at the back of my neck at the feeling of him watching me do so. I wonder if he's going to be like this all day. I know I should have saved the original presentation somewhere else, I think to myself, but it was an honest mistake.

I open up a fresh PowerPoint page and we begin, trying to remember which graphs we included and the order of the slides. He gets frustrated when I can't find the font we used for the headings, something I think is ridiculously pedantic. Because I'm not trying to find the one he likes, he places his hand over mine on the mouse so he can force the arrow to hover over the toolbar. I'm momentarily distracted by how childish he's being because his hand on mine is so firm, so commanding. When he makes my finger push down on the left button the thrill of it rushes down into my pants.

Then he goes back to being a dickhead, sending me out to buy us lunch but not saying thank you for it, telling me how slow I'm being, gleefully pointing out my spelling mistakes. As the light fades outside, I announce I need the loo. I don't, but I need to stretch my legs, to get away from him.

'You can go when we're done with this slide,' he says, hovering over me sitting in the chair.

That's the final straw. 'Why are you being so rude to me?' I snap. 'I didn't mean to lose the presentation. Maybe if you didn't always make me print everything out for you I would have emailed it to you, and then you'd have had it on file – did you think of that?'

The air in his big, empty office rings with my words like a bell's just chimed. He doesn't say a word, he simply stares at me, his face abruptly close to mine. Panic floods through me – fuck, I just shouted at my boss.

Then, ever so slightly, he smiles. I think he might be impressed. 'You're right,' he says. 'I'm sorry.' I'm so shocked that my words worked, I don't know what to do next. 'Let's take a break.' He goes over to a cupboard by the door, pulls out a bottle of wine and two tumblers. The bottle lid cracks pleasingly as he opens it, followed by the glug, glug, glug of the liquid as it hits the glasses and an aroma of sweet oakiness fills the room. As he hands me one, he holds my stare and my pussy begins to feel hot.

'To you,' he says, not taking his eyes off me as he clinks his glass

against the one I'm holding. 'Thank you for your hard work today.'
I narrow my eyes as I take a gulp. 'What's that look for?' he says.

'You sounded a little sarcastic,' I reply.

He laughs. 'I can't win with you,' he says, taking a sip. He has a
bead of wine on his lip. I know I'm being transparent, but I can't
help but gaze longingly at it as he wipes it away. 'You stare at me a lot,
did you know that?'

My cheeks flush, betraying me, but at least he can't see my pussy.
If he could, he'd know it was throbbing, swelling against my knickers
all because he's looking at me so intently. I don't say anything. He
comes to sit on the edge of the desk right next to me and my heart
begins to pound with anticipation. 'I promise that I'm sorry, and that
I'm grateful for your hard work – not just today, but all this week.'

'Okay.' I nod, believing him.

With a small, goading smile he adds, 'But I am a little mad at
you, yes.'

I bite my lip. Swallow. 'What can I do to make it up to you?' I say.
I know what I want him to ask of me. I'm daring him to ask it.

Quietly, without breaking eye contact, he says, 'You can get up,
you can bend over this desk, and you can pull up your dress and let
me spank you.'

I'm breathing so shallowly I feel light-headed. The wetness from
my pussy is soaking into my knickers. I get up from the chair and
I do as he says. The rush of cool air on the back of my legs feels
tantalising. My forehead is resting on my hands, which I've placed
on the desk. I hear his slow, deliberate footsteps as he moves around

behind me. He yanks my knickers up into the folds of my pussy to reveal my butt cheeks. I know he must be able to see how wet the material is. Then I wait.

The sting of his hand as it meets my cheek feels so good, so necessary, that I let out a moan. The frustration that has been building all day wasn't just about work; it was sexual all along. He slaps the other cheek, his hand lingering there afterwards, applying pressure to the sharp, hot pain that's so pleasurable to me. He does it twice more: slap, sting, press; slap, sting, press. I imagine the handprints that are forming, as if I've been branded by him.

'Get up,' he says. I do, turning to face him. 'I'm still a little mad at you.'

My eyelids flutter, my whole body seems to tremble. 'I'll do anything you want me to,' I say.

'Will you put my cock in your mouth?' he asks. I nod. 'Get down on your knees.'

He unzips the jeans he's wearing and his cock springs out. It's long, smooth and girthy. I open my mouth obediently, and he fills it. It's exactly what I want. I feel greed rumble down inside me as my tongue explores his shaft, as he runs his hands through my hair, keeping my head firmly in place, as saliva fills my mouth hungrily around his smooth, warm, pulsating cock. He is moaning now; I feel triumphant – I'm doing that to him.

He pulls out of me suddenly, his hands still in my hair. 'Will you still do anything?' he says, looking down at me on my knees by his feet.

'Yes,' I breathe.

He tells me to take off my dress and my pants and go to the window. I do as I'm told, the thrill of danger tingling over me as I survey the darkening city and twinkling lights that are spread out before me, wondering if anybody in the nearby offices can see me. I hear the tell-tale tear of a packet and then feel his breath on my shoulder. He unhooks my bra and the straps tickle my arms as they fall down. He presses me, totally naked, firmly against the glass. The coldness bites pleasurably at my nipples and my belly. I feel so turned on, my pussy throbbing so achingly that I think I might shatter.

I love that I'm naked and that he's fully dressed with only his condomed cock out. He teases my bare butt with it. 'Spread your legs,' he whispers into my ear. I do it. With no warning, he plunges inside me. I feel the firm length of him glide easily in and out because I'm maybe the wettest I've ever been in my life. The thought that people might be watching us makes my heart beat faster and my thirst for him heavier. My moans beg him to fuck me harder and he obeys. He leans one hand on the glass as he pumps; I put my hand over his and tense my pussy muscles, staring down at the lights of the cars thirty floors below, the fear of being so high up adding to the intensity of my pleasure. His cock rocks inside me, filling me hungrily. I reach down to my clit, brushing it back and forth, my pussy gripping harder on to him.

It's getting too much; I can feel myself reaching my limits and my legs start shaking. **As I cum, he fucks me harder and harder and I scream out in ecstasy as he groans throatily himself, cumming in**

spasms inside me, shuddering to a standstill.

I lean my forehead against the cool glass.

He bites my ear gently, his breath heavy from the exercise. 'Now I've forgiven you,' he says.

TIP 7:

INDIRECT CLIT ACTION

There are so many ways to touch yourself and really you can be the artist, there are no rules. If you're looking for some inspiration, however, I have your back.

Earlier we mentioned just how many nerve endings are in your clitoris, so we know that this can be a very sensitive area. Sometimes directly stimulating your clit can be too much, so there are ways we can indirectly touch it instead. Even if you like direct clit action, why not give these two ideas a go in the next meditation and see what you think of them.

THE BURGER

Take two fingers on each hand to either side of your outer labia and press together in a way that sandwiches your clitoris inside. Then move one of your hands up and down while keeping the other one still to start creating an indirect rub on your clitoris. This technique could be easier with less lube so that you have the friction to keep your fingers in place. Experiment with up and down, back and forth, and circular motions.

TEASE

Use one or two fingers and a bit of lube to trace around your clitoris and your labia. This technique enables you to find which parts of your vulva you find most sensitive. Explore with lighter and firm touches and rubbing in circular, stroking, figure of eights, or back and forth motions. One movement in particular could be orbiting around the clitoris over and over again.

EX SEX

READING TIME

<10 MINUTES

THE SEXUAL PARTNER IS

FIRM AND FAMILIAR

SEXY CHECKLIST

☐ MASTURBATION
☐ CLIT PLAY/FINGERING
☐ CUNNILINGUS
☐ BLOW JOB
☐ NIPPLE PLAY
■ VAGINAL PENETRATION
☐ ANAL/BUTT PLAY
☐ SPANKING
☐ SEX TOYS
■ CHOKING
☐ BDSM

I'm sardined on a commuter train at 6 p.m. between various sweaty armpits. As the train slows and speeds up again we are all swaying together in one big blob of bodies. I gaze, absent-mindedly, over the various different heads in the carriage when one in particular catches my eye. I stare at the back of a man's head. No . . . it can't be. His hair bounces slightly with the train, the early-evening light slicing through the windows making it shine.

The train stops and a few people squeeze themselves out on to the platform. He readjusts himself. Now he's looking towards me. Our eyes catch each other's at the exact same time. My ex-boyfriend. The one that got away. I feel a flutter in my stomach, my heart feels as if it's kicking against my chest. I let my eyes roam that face I used to hold so close to my own, his arm that's holding on to the rails but used to wrap around me on cold nights and in hot beds. Fuck.

The train comes to a stop again. I realise this is my stop and, panicked, I grab my bag, which is by my feet. I look back up and he is gone. Feeling flustered, wondering if maybe I'd just daydreamed that whole scene, I practically fall through the doors just in time.

'Let me . . . ' There he is, holding out his hand to steady me. I feel my breath catch in my throat, butterflies in a flurry of activity in my stomach. He's smiling at me. Even though I've already steadied myself, I take his hand instinctively and it's as if electricity prickles at my fingers as I do.

'Um, hi,' I manage, quickly removing my hand from his and slinging my bag over my shoulder.

'Hey,' he says, still smiling. We stand in the middle of the bustling platform locked in this strange moment. It feels familiar and completely different all at the same time. People move around us but we just stand here looking at each other. I realise I should probably ask him the basic catch-up questions.

'It's been a while,' I say. 'How have you been?'

'I've been great actually. Me and Freya . . . ' He eyes me carefully. 'We've just moved into a new place, it's nice. I . . . ah . . . So how are things with you?'

I'd heard about this girlfriend before, but my stomach still somersaults when he says her name. Even when we've moved on ourselves, why does it feel so human to want the people we once loved to stay in love with us?

'Yeah, I'm great too.' Mimicking his words, I summarise my recent history. My current boyfriend and I have just been away to Mexico together and had the best time. My ex smiles as I tell him; I know he is relieved I'm happy, too. But did his stomach somersault when I said my boyfriend's name? Am I mean for hoping it did?

People are still walking down the platform and someone accidentally jostles him. 'Hey, do you fancy taking this off the platform? It would be great to catch up some more.'

He seems properly genuine, his eyes wide and round, almost sparkling with hope.

'Okay,' I hear myself saying. 'Maybe we could go to the bar. You know, The—' He cuts me off.

'Of course I remember our bar. Let's do it.'

We walk towards one of our old haunts. I wonder whether this is a good idea or not; the sparks I felt at the touch of his hand, the somersault when I heard his girlfriend's name . . . There's a tension in the air between us, something unfinished. I wonder how my boyfriend would feel if he knew I was going for drinks spontaneously with my ex. What would Freya think? Both of them completely unaware of what we're up to . . . But maybe I'm reading too much into this. It's just a friendly catch-up with an old friend.

An old friend I used to have mind-blowing sex with.

We sit where we always used to sit, the waitress we recognise still serving drinks, the cosy selection of odd chairs and dim amber lighting. We order the same drinks. I twist my straw in the glass, the ice tinkling on the sides. He's looking so intently at me, with such a warm, well-meaning smile.

I purposely talk about mundane things to try to dispel the tension, but even that's so comfortable and easy that it feels exciting. We order another round. Mundane chat turns to light teasing. My cheeks start to feel hot, either from the alcohol or from the flirtatiousness of our conversation. Our eye contact is hardly breaking, he doesn't even look when he puts his glass down; it catches on the vase that's on the table and falls over, shooting the last of his drink across the surface. We both rush to mop it up with napkins – and our fingers touch. A wave of memories seems to be erupting on my skin. The last time we had sex, the first time he kissed me, the way he used to stroke my hair, massage my neck. He looks up at me with an expression that tells me he felt it too. A longing in his eyes mirroring my own. I have this feeling of temptation washing over me, travelling up my gut and into my throat. It's too much.

'I need the loo.' I push back my chair and basically run into the dark corridor of the bar to the bathroom. My heart is beating out of my chest, thumping against my ribcage. I need to escape the intensity of the situation at the table. I stare at myself in the mirror. Remind myself that my boyfriend is at home waiting for me, probably making dinner for the two of us. I gather myself to walk back to the table and tell my ex that I need to leave.

I turn the handle. I know before I pull it open what I'll find there.

He's standing right outside, with an almost desperate look on his face, his chest rising and falling noticeably. God, I'm so glad; I wanted him to be there, I wanted him to be there so fucking badly. He takes my shoulders and pushes me back into the bathroom, locking the door behind us. Before I can stop to think about what happens next he leans down and kisses me hard on the lips. It lingers, a warm magnetic kiss. A kiss I hate to say I've missed.

He pulls back from me, running the back of his hand over his open mouth and looking at me as if he can't believe he just did that. 'I'm sorry,' he says. 'I shouldn't have done that.' He goes to put his hand on the door handle but I can't let him go. I put a flat palm to the door, not looking at him. If I look at him, I know what I'll do.

And then he says my name. Quietly but luxuriously. And it seems to speak to something deep inside me. I grab his face in my hands and slip my tongue into his mouth. He falls into me, giving me everything back, his hands roaming around my body, reclaiming me. Our breath is loud and intense. The kiss is hungry and passionate.

He pushes me against the wall and I feel his huge erection pressing into me. My pussy throbs at the memory of what he feels like inside. He kisses down my neck, sending shivers of pleasure along my spine. I grapple with his jeans, unbuttoning him and pushing them down. He pulls his briefs off, his cock springing to life. I reach under my dress and pull my own knickers down and kick them off my feet. For a second we stand there taking in the moment, how wrong what we're doing is.

He spits on his fingers and pulls up my dress, passing them down over my extremely ready pussy. He moans as he feels me again.

'Fuck, I've missed you,' he says.

I run my thumb over his lips; I never thought I'd be this near them again. 'I've missed you too.'

And with that he pushes his cock into me as he presses me against the wall, edging in slowly, letting me revel in the memories. Holy shit. I forgot just how perfect he feels. I gasp as he thrusts deeper into me.

'You feel so fucking amazing,' he groans.

My hands search his body, holding on to him as hard as I can, as he moves himself in and out of my dripping-wet pussy. Every time he pushes deeper into me a wave of pleasure rolls through, growing inside of me and crashing, releasing in moans from my lips. His cock hits my G-spot so perfectly, every motion sending me into euphoria.

'We shouldn't be doing this,' I breathe into his ear.

He fucks me harder. He takes his hand to my throat, controlling me, as if I couldn't get more turned on as it is. My breath is held by his hand, searching for air but also not needing it at the same time.

He loosens his grip and I inhale sharply, catching my breath, pleasure swirling through me as I feed myself with oxygen again.

His cheek is pressed against mine, warm and soft. 'Your pussy is the best I've ever had,' he says into my ear as he plunges in and out. I never knew I needed to hear those words until he said them. It's as if he's rubbed my clit with them, as if I can feel them inside my hot, wet pussy.

'I've missed your dick so much,' I respond, pulling him into me, and he thanks me by plunging in deeper and pulling out slowly – letting me feel his whole length and girth. I can feel every centimetre of his cock brushing through me and I whimper with the pleasure, heartbroken at not having this feeling in my life any more, at how bad I'm being, at how fucking good this feels.

We lock in an embrace, two bodies completely melting into one as our pleasure reaches its climax. **Trembling, my body collapses into him as I reach orgasm, his hand moving to cover my loud moans. My pussy constricts around him, my head swimming, light from the surge of energy.**

He cums inside me, his body shuddering to stillness, and we stand pressed up against the wall. Sweaty and confused. He moves his hand away from my mouth and replaces it with a deep kiss, leaning our foreheads together, breathing in an old flame.

We gather ourselves, walk back to the table one by one. We sit down and finish our drinks, pay, and at the front door we say goodbye. We walk in different directions.

I look back as he walks away, and he turns to watch me too.

TIP 8:

DIRECT CLIT ACTION

For some, direct stimulation might be the golden pathway to euphoria, so let's go through some techniques you could bring in while you're reading the next meditation. If your clit feels too sensitive to touch directly, you might want to try them out over fabric – like knickers or bed sheets. But definitely don't do it if you know direct touching isn't for you – instead, I would suggest you use the next story to explore any and all parts of your body, like I mentioned on page 32.

You can use these techniques just above your clit so you're still on the hood or you can pull back and directly touch the clit head (this is why getting to know your anatomy is so useful!):

DJ

We joke about this being the way guys try to pleasure us (you might have seen the TikToks), but if used properly this can actually be an effective technique. Use three or more fingers flat together and rub back and forth or in circular motions over your clitoris. This works particularly well in combination with lubricant. You can speed up or slow down the motion and change the amount of pressure you're applying depending on what's feeling good.

JOYSTICK

Using one or two fingers you rub on the clit or the clit hood with an up-and-down, side-to-side or circular motion. You can change up the pace and pressure, fast or slow, hard or soft. Again, this works really well when it's wet – the more lube the better!

FIGURE OF EIGHT

Like the above, using lube and a finger or two, work your way around in a figure of eight. You can change up the pressure and speed in certain loops. Also figure out the placement of the eight that works for you. Are you circling around the clit or going over it?

Most direct clitoral techniques involve fingers, vibrators or the rubbing of various objects, and it really is about finding what works for you. Your key things to notice in your exploration are: pressure, speed and movement style. I would suggest you go rogue and freestyle once you have these basic techniques. Mix and match, widen your circles or strokes or minimise them, tap lightly, press firmly, go super slowly, speed it up – try it all out.

NOTE: While I've said above 'speed it up', sometimes faster is not better if you're looking for orgasm – often you can build bigger pleasure by going slow and steady. Most people's pleasure loves rhythm and consistency, so sometimes using too much of a variety of techniques can delay orgasm or lose it completely. Repetitive movements with a good solid rhythm are often the most 'foolproof' – so if you're up for mixing and matching, don't go so far with it that you frustrate yourself.

MY BOYFRIEND AND HER

READING TIME

<7 MINUTES

THE SEXUAL PARTNERS ARE

OPEN-MINDED AND SEXY

SEXY CHECKLIST

■ MASTURBATION
■ CLIT PLAY/FINGERING
■ CUNNILINGUS
■ BLOW JOB
■ NIPPLE PLAY
■ VAGINAL PENETRATION
□ ANAL/BUTT PLAY
□ SPANKING
■ SEX TOYS
□ CHOKING
□ BDSM

The warm hum of voices teases my ears as I swing my feet from a tall stool, waiting for my boyfriend to arrive. It's a dark, moody set-up, with orange lights underneath the bar creating a sexy, sensual vibe – which is exactly why we picked it.

I've always been curious about open relationships. How would it feel if my boyfriend fucked another woman? The thought has been turning around my mind a lot lately, having morphed into: what if he fucked another woman . . . while I watched? I think about watching him with someone else when I masturbate. Him looking over to me while he has his cock in her pussy, as she moans loudly because he feels so good inside her. I know how good he could make her feel. His cock is the best cock I've ever had the privilege of having in me; it seems a shame to keep it all to myself. It's big, and slightly curved, which we all know hits the exact right spot.

There's a squeeze on my shoulder sending a glorious shiver down my spine. My boyfriend is looking down at me, greeting me with a kiss and a smile before he slips into the seat beside me. He swallows nervously but his eyes are wide and alert. He's excited.

It's only a couple of minutes later that we see her. She's taken a seat on the other side of the bar, leaning on it with effortless seduction so that we can see the top of her breasts, her hand tracing the rim of her drink, her lips pouted slightly. My boyfriend and I look at each other. I take a deep breath and nod. He takes my hand in his and we walk over to her to say hello, both our hearts thumping in our throats.

She's expecting us. This is a chemistry meeting. If all goes well, we could all be going home with each other tonight. She stands up to say hello, her bum grazing the bar stool as she does so. She's Insta-famous beautiful, wearing a dress that follows her curves. She hugs me and I smell her perfume: it's sweet and delicious. Then she hugs my boyfriend. My pussy pulses.

'You look really hot together,' I say before I can stop myself.

My boyfriend smiles a little awkwardly, but she laughs easily, brushing her hair back with a hand. She looks at him and then back at me. Licking her lips slightly, she says, 'You're a very lucky woman.' I'm sold.

Half an hour later and we're all squished in the back seat of a taxi. She's in the middle – her bare thighs are pressed against my boyfriend's and mine. She takes one of my hands in hers and then does the same to him and places them in her warm lap. It's as if an electric energy is radiating through our bodies.

I want to tell my boyfriend to kiss her, but I don't want the taxi driver to hear. I catch my boyfriend's eye and mouth it instead. He raises his eyebrows. This will be the first step down the rabbit hole. Who knows what will happen after this? He takes a deep breath and then leans forward, tilting her chin to face him with his finger, and locks her into a deep kiss. Fuck. I feel the lips of my pussy swelling.

I lead her from our front door up to our bedroom. I sit with my back against the pillows – they both sit on the end of the bed, close to each other. My boyfriend looks at me to check I'm definitely sure I want him to do this. I nod hungrily at him. I don't just *want* him to touch her now; I *need* him to touch her. He swallows and says to her:

'Undress for me.'

She stands and obliges. His eyes never leave her as she ever so slowly pushes each strap of her dress from her shoulders and lets it fall mesmerisingly to the ground. She's wearing a strapless red lacy bra and matching panties. The hunger in his eyes as he surveys her almost-naked body excites me in a way I've never felt before. I'm excited for him.

She slowly reaches behind her back and unhooks her bra. Her breasts spring free from the cups and her nipples immediately contract. She flings the bra away and walks forward until her crotch is immediately in his face. He grabs her ass and squeezes her into him, inhaling her scent. He's finding this so easy, and I'm finding that so hot.

He pulls down her knickers. Then he kisses around her thighs, making her moan gently as he teases her. I feel saliva pooling in my mouth as I watch my boyfriend kiss her pussy. He slips a tongue around her clit and traces a hand up between her legs, plunging two fingers inside her. She gasps at the immediate pleasure as he rhythmically pulses inside her.

I'm so aroused that I can't bear it any more; I reach down to my bedside table drawer and pull out a small vibrator. I push aside my own knickers and place the vibrator between my legs. My body is rippling with desire, lust and pleasure. My boyfriend looks at me. 'What should I do next to her?' he says. He's not out of his own ideas; he just knows I love to give commands.

'Touch her breasts,' I say.

He runs his hands firmly up her waist to her breasts and cups them, running his fingers lightly over her hard nipples in a way that clearly tickles her in just the right way, because she swallows and grabs hold of his shoulders, her fingers digging into his skin. Then she pushes him down on to the bed and straddles him. He quickly unbuckles between her legs and pulls his erect cock out of his pants. Seeing her eyes widen at my boyfriend's cock sends tremors around my clit as I touch my vibrator closely to myself. I hold my breath in anticipation of seeing him penetrate her.

'Fuck, you're a big boy,' she says, her eyes twinkling longingly. She backs off him so she can lean down and take him into her mouth. I can't help but moan quietly behind them as she sucks his cock, taking it deep into her throat.

My boyfriend reaches his hand out to me, beckoning me over. I crawl towards him and lock him in a deeply passionate, upside-down kiss as he moans into my mouth. I look down at her – the fact I'm kissing him while she has his cock in her mouth makes me want to cry out with pleasure.

I stop kissing him abruptly because I want them to continue just the two of them. As if she's heard me think that, she stops sucking him, gets up and goes round to the other side of the bed to me, climbing on and resting her head on the pillow so that she's facing me. I watch the way her breasts pool together on the arm beneath her, how it makes the curve of her hip, ass and waist more obvious. My boyfriend, confused at where she's gone, sits up.

'Get behind me,' she tells him. 'I want you like this.'

Before he does as she says, he reaches to the bedside drawer and pulls out a condom, tearing the wrapper quickly and sliding it down the curve of his cock. He spoons her, tucking her hair out of the way, running his hand lightly down the length of her arm. They both look straight at me as he penetrates her.

'Fuck,' she moans as he fills her, her eyes still stuck on mine. I know how he feels inside, I know how good it is and what she must be feeling, which makes it all the more orgasmic to watch. I look at my boyfriend – he's grabbing on to her arse, closing his eyes now, biting his lip. I work my vibrator around my clit in circles, pressing rhythmically on it. My eyes roll back in my head as it sends me so close to the edge – but I bring myself back into the room because it's watching them moving together, my boyfriend's skilful thrusts and the way her breasts ripple as he expends them, on top of the sounds of them moaning and the smell of their sex, that's doing it for me. I can't stop watching how hot he looks while fucking, having never seen him from this view before. The way his arm and his stomach muscles are tensing pleasingly as his cock continues to draw out of her before sinking back into her. I watch him edging close, his face contorting in concentration, the look I know all too well. He opens his eyes and looks at me as he plunges into her again and again, eliciting whimpers of pleasure from her. I move the vibrator more vigorously on myself, building my own orgasm. **Him cumming, pulsing inside her, and her moans at the feel of it sends me spiralling into my own climax. I writhe on the bed, my eyes still open looking at the two of them together: my boyfriend and her.**

We lie there panting. She holds an arm out to me and I wriggle over to her, pressing myself up against her naked body, feeling the warmth of her soft parts against me and the wetness of her pussy on my bare leg. From behind her my boyfriend reaches out his hand and strokes my face. Will anything ever be this hot again?

TIP 9:

WHAT TO DO WHEN NOTHING'S 'WORKING'

Sometimes masturbating doesn't do anything for us and that's likely either because we're not in the right brain space or because we've been too dismissive of our turn ons or turn offs (see page 22). But sometimes, it's doing *something* that isn't really going anywhere, or we're really close to the edge but it's just not happening. This could be because we're chasing the orgasm too hard and getting frustrated, so our bodies are becoming tense, or just because in general we're not relaxed enough; our minds are connecting up with our bodies.

If this ever happens to you – you feel frustrated and as if nothing is working – then I'd like to suggest three things.

1. Use the simple breathing technique on page 56 – either in conjunction with touching yourself or take your hands off until you're feeling completely relaxed.

2. Take your hands away from your vulva and start caressing your body instead for a few moments to reset.

3. Give yourself a belly rub. This might sound weird but bear with me! Sometimes you need to refocus and reframe in your session. One of the most random things I've discovered on my own journey is that if I breathe deeply and rub my hands around my stomach in a circular motion just above my pubic mount, the pleasure starts to regrow and I'm able to

rebuild. This technique works especially well if you're using a vibrator. One hand holds the vibrations to your clit and the other massages your belly in a circular motion. I'm no scientist, but this really helps your mind focus on the sensations that are happening in your pelvic region and gets you out of your mind! Why not try this halfway through the next masturbation meditation even if your climax is 'working', to slow things down? When you start directly touching yourself again, it might help you to really connect with your pleasure in new ways.

LUXURY LUST

READING TIME
<7 MINUTES

THE SEXUAL PARTNER IS
RICH

SEXY CHECKLIST
☐ MASTURBATION
■ CLIT PLAY/FINGERING
■ CUNNILINGUS
☐ BLOW JOB
☐ NIPPLE PLAY
■ VAGINAL PENETRATION
☐ ANAL/BUTT PLAY
☐ SPANKING
☐ SEX TOYS
☐ CHOKING
☐ BDSM

He takes my hand. I feel the warmth of his palm press against mine; his skin isn't soft, but it's smooth and firm.

I step out of the car – a sleek black car he sent to pick me up, something that's definitely never happened to me before. I'm wearing a black dress with a halter neckline and the cold night air licks pleasantly at my bare shoulders. Something about being around him makes all my senses heightened.

He leads me into the restaurant.

The people around us look up as we pass. How can they not? My date, Eric, has the features of a modern Viking: strong jawline, a defined nose, bright but narrow eyes that make him seem all-knowing. He is suited and booted, his luxury shirt is stretched taut against his muscular frame and he smells expensive: vanilla, a hint of cedarwood.

We're seated at a cosy corner booth. He rests his elbows on the white tablecloth and clasps his hands together, looks straight at me with those narrow eyes so that I'm transfixed. He asks me what I thought about the gallery – where we met – and suddenly we fall through a trapdoor into deep chat, about everything and nothing at the same time. He feels like a castle with never-ending rooms full of interesting ideas and secrets that I want to explore; as soon as I'm in one I'm impatient to get to the next. His voice is soft and deep, words seem to strum it.

The waiter comes over multiple times to see if we're ready to order. Eventually, without glancing at the menu, Eric says we'll try the lobster and caviar. I've never eaten either before. How many new tastes will I have tonight? The food melts in my mouth. Under the table his leg brushes mine unintentionally. I feel like a fox spotted in the middle of the road: alert, waiting for more movement.

Time moves quickly and I am back in the sleek black car, this time with him next to me. He takes my hand and moves it up to his mouth, firmly kisses the back of it. The touch of skin, his lips on me, shoots shivers up my arm and down my spine. He wraps an arm around my bare shoulder and pulls me to his side. Up close I smell leather and something smoky, as if he literally just walked out of an old novel. I can hear his heart beating, a slow steady drum.

Calmly, he takes my chin between his thumb and forefinger and tilts my face up to look at him. I want to run my tongue over that hard, square jaw, I think. Then he leans down and kisses me, not the soft first kiss that I expected, but passionately, exploratively, his tongue deep inside my mouth. It slows down; now it's twirling around mine, tasting me, and I'm tasting him. The hand that tilted up my chin moves down to hold my neck and my heartbeat quickens. If before I felt like a fox, now I feel like a vulnerable young rabbit in his bloodlust Viking grip. His kiss takes on a deeper hunger – but we're interrupted. The car has stopped. I let out a small moan of frustration. He laughs softly.

We've pulled up to an old, grand house, ghostly pale between large trees that dapple the street lights. Eric sweeps out of the car; I can see him moving round to my side, to open the door for me. My heart pounds. Just like earlier, he takes my hand and I step into the cold night air.

He opens the front door of the house into a dimly lit, echoey entrance hall, our shoes clipping against the floor tiles. Wrapped around the vast walls is an impressive, wide staircase, golden banisters shimmering in the light from a twinkling chandelier above. I knew he must be rich but I wasn't expecting this.

He leads me by the hand up the stairs, slowing down outside a large eggshell-white door and turns to me. In one swift movement he scoops me up into his arms and pushes the door open with a sharp kick. As my eyes adjust to the almost-darkness I see that we're in a modern, sleek bedroom, at odds with the rest of the old house. He places me on the low, king-sized bed. The mattress gives underneath me and I can feel the luxurious softness of his expensive sheets; they slip under my hands as I steady myself. I realise we haven't spoken a word since the restaurant – our lips and hands have taken over the talking. The silence between us has gained a tangible energy, a palpable pull between our bodies.

He stands back and begins to undress slowly in front of me.

Carefully undoing his shirt one button at a time.

Dropping it to the floor, the mess looking like a piece of art in the clean room.

He unbuckles his belt, the clink of the metal piercing the sound of the room. The leather stretching from the trouser loops, the brush of the thick strap between his hands and the thud as it also lands on the floor.

My lips part and I can feel the saliva filling around my tongue as I watch him. The muscles on his torso catch the light from the lamps outside the window. I am desperate to run my hands over the shadows their definitions create but he is in charge here.

Now he steps out of his trousers and is left standing there in tight briefs that leave nothing to the imagination.

Coming closer he stands in front of me so that his hard cock, pressing through the material, is right in front of my face. My nerves tingle at the back of my throat at the excitement of seeing him fully. I take hold of his briefs and pull down; his cock springs out, ready and standing to attention. I look up at him and he nods at me.

I take his hard cock in my hands, but just as I'm about to put my mouth around it, he grabs me and pushes me back on to the bed. My heart skips a beat, thumping with adrenalin at the change in plan. He pulls at my clothes, and I help him ease me out of them until all that's left are my lace knickers. He pulls them carefully down my thighs and calves and they drop to the floor with the sound of a sigh. His eyes rove over my nakedness, over the parts he hasn't yet seen, lingering on my nipples and the curves of my hips.

He uses his knees to spread my legs. My breath is heavy, my pussy tingling, desperate for touch.

He begins by my feet. I close my eyes and fall into the moment, his lips teasing up my smooth legs and up my inner thighs, kissing, licking and biting softly. He's so close, yet so far away. My pulse quickens loudly, as if my ears are speakers rumbling with the bass. His hands reach around and squeeze my bum cheeks. He pulls me towards him and kisses me deeply on my pussy. His tongue swirling and sucking on my clit, running up and down the inside of my labia with firm, hot strokes. I feel a heat rising through my entire body, flushing my cheeks and my chest. My hands grab on to his hair and hold him on to me.

He pushes two fingers inside me and I realise how wet I am. I sharply inhale at the first penetration. Moans start to escape me, and he moans too, humming deeply into me, creating a vibration sensation. I tremble from the sound radiating into my skin; it sends shivers across my thighs.

I'm beginning to climax, but then he stops and sits up. I look down and see his dick ready to be inside me. He tears open a condom packet and with one fluid motion gracefully pulls the condom on to it. He leans over me so we're groin to groin, face to face, kissing me deeply, his tongue filling up my mouth. He teases the entrance to my wet pussy with his fingers and then – he pushes his cock deep inside of me. As he thrusts into me he bites on my lip, feeling my moan of pleasure fill his own mouth.

With each push and pull of his hips, flickers of electricity shoot through my pussy and up into my head. My eyes are searching for something to hold. My hands claw at his back and he growls from the depths of his throat. I bite on to his shoulder as he presses on my G-spot, each moment feeling like I'm losing my grip on reality. He takes hold of my hands and pulls them above my head, holding me down, unmoving in his control.

His grip tenses and the rhythm of his hips becomes more controlled, an energy building between us taking us to the brink of orgasm. I wrap my legs around his back. He pushes himself deep inside, curves back up, then again, again, again. I open my eyes and look at his beautiful Viking face. We're both on the edge, staring into each other's eyes, making a pact to jump off together. And then –

We climax simultaneously, my moans entangled with his groans as the weight of his damp, muscular body blankets mine.

We both lie there, wet with our own sweat and fluids, holding on to each other. Our chests rise and fall with our breath, trying to regain a natural flow. He squeezes me tightly, scattering kisses over my forehead and face, before we both melt off into a satisfied sleep.

TIP 10:

INVEST IN SEX TOYS

Try sex toys. Please, *please* try them.

This might sound like an obvious one to some, but you'd be surprised how many people don't explore any of the sex toy market. A lot of people think they shouldn't need to use sex toys, that if they do it means that they are broken or lacking in some way. That couldn't be further from the truth! I would guess that some of the reasons we think this are: for years in movies and porn we have seen women cumming easily from penetration, making it seem like that kind of sex, without sex toys, was the norm. Partners have typically feared sex toys, feeling like they will replace them. Sex education never taught us about female pleasure, and that's what so many sex toys are specifically created for. Sometimes, the way sex toys are marketed, it feels like they're just for the sexually adventurous, the kink community, swingers. I just have one thing to say to all this: sex toys are for you, too.

If you're starting at the bottom, or the bare bedside drawer in this case, there is an extremely large selection of toys out there and it can be overwhelming. You might be wondering where to start, or what's going to work for you and your body. So let's think about the way you already know you like to pleasure yourself. Do you love clitoral stimulation? If you do, you might want to start with the very basic bullet vibrator. This was the first ever sex toy I owned and it was the perfect beginner's toy. It's small, discreet, quiet and it kind of acts as your finger, if your finger vibrated at a super speed. Another great thing about these toys is that they're the most reasonably priced when you're just dipping your toe in for the first time.

Do you really enjoy penetration? If yes, you might want to explore G-spot stimulators. These are insertable toys and some come with a vibration function. The vibrations can be extremely pleasurable although not everyone feels them the same inside. You can also get lovely glass dildos or something that looks more penis-like – both give you that 'fullness' feeling which might suit you better if you're not sensitive to internal vibrations.

Are you a huge fan of oral sex? Genius toy inventors have created clit suction technology! This toy looks a little like medical apparatus (in a cool way), and creates a small air compression around your clit when there is skin contact. The suction feeling on your clit mimics . . . well, sucking! It's mind blowing, trust me.

Do you like clitoral stimulation and penetration at the same time? Then a dual-pleasure vibrator is the one for you. These are insertable vibrators that have an outer part that fits over your clit for maximum pleasure! These always drive me wild, and are definitely a must-have in my bedside drawer. On that note, in case it's useful for you to see an example of what a fun bedside table can look like, here are my personal essentials:

- Small clitoral vibrator – for exploring my vulva and clitoris

- Rabbit/dual-pleasure vibrator – when I want to fully indulge in all sensations

- Wand vibrator – my go-to full-power toy for insane clitoral stimulation

- Lube (water based for use with toys and condoms)

- Oil for self-massage

Sex toys are very exciting when it comes to enhancing your pleasure. But a word of caution: sometimes they make it too bloody easy. To make the most of your sex toys, take your time, use lube and experiment with the settings the toy comes with (if any). It's also worth trying your toys in different positions and locations. Many toys are waterproof (always check the label) and make a great addition to a relaxing bath time. Use the lower settings on your vibrator to build up the pleasure slowly. Lastly, try taking the toys away just before you cum to create a longer, bigger climax – also see my tip on edging (page 176).

NOTE: Make sure you invest in good-quality products made of body-safe materials, such as medical-grade silicone. If you are unsure, check with a shop assistant or customer services. Avoid jelly, rubber or lesser-grade silicones, as these materials could be harmful to your body and pH balance.

BEING WATCHED

READING TIME
<7 MINUTES

THE SEXUAL PARTNER IS
FEMININE

SEXY CHECKLIST
■ MASTURBATION
■ CLIT PLAY/FINGERING
☐ CUNNILINGUS
☐ BLOW JOB
■ NIPPLE PLAY
■ VAGINAL PENETRATION
☐ ANAL/BUTT PLAY
☐ SPANKING
■ SEX TOYS
☐ CHOKING
☐ BDSM

I look out of my floor-to-ceiling window as I undress for a shower. I half notice the bustle of life on the narrow street way below – and my neighbour sitting in her bedroom opposite mine, twenty feet away. It's funny how living in a high-rise gives you such an insight into the buildings opposite. I probably see more of these people going about their daily lives than I do my friends. I often catch glimpses of this neighbour in particular as she gets changed in the mornings. I don't look on purpose, but it's hard not to. I find her body . . . beguiling, especially her breasts – she has nipples that always appear hard – and her bush, which she leaves natural.

I'm naked now, so I grab my towel and leave my room for the shower, unaware that I, too, might be being watched.

I re-enter my bedroom, smelling sweet from my moisturiser – and my skin suddenly tingles; it's that inexplicable feeling that somebody's looking at you. I instinctively glance out of my long window and – startled – see that my neighbour is still in her room. She's sitting on her bed with her legs crossed in front of her own window, in a thin, pale pink, silk robe, and she's staring directly at me. A surge of adrenalin washes over me. I must have seen her a hundred times but our eyes have never locked on each other before. I stand stock-still, watching her back, unable to move. She smiles. My heart begins to thump. Does her smile simply mean 'hello', or does it mean something else?

As if in answer to my question, she bites her lip seductively. She's flirting with me. I'm suddenly more aware of my naked body under my towel; excitement floods through me and I can feel a pulse fluttering in my pussy. Her eyes leave mine to move down, slowly, over my towel, as if she's asking me to take it off. I have the urge to accept, to let it fall to the floor and expose myself to her. She might not be asking for that, of course. If I've got it wrong, then I will be so embarrassed I'll have to move out. Her eyes come back up to mine, she tilts her head to one side and raises her eyebrows. Her expression is definitely expectant, almost impatient. Thump, thump, thump, goes my pussy. I take a deep breath in and exhale a deep breath out.

I drop the towel.

Her eyes start at my feet and trace my calves and my thighs, rove over the mound above my pussy, my stomach and my waist, until she stops on my breasts. I automatically move my hands to cup them, unsure of what I'm doing, of what to do next. But the excitement is now trembling between the lips of my pussy. My breasts weigh in my palms, feeling soft and supple against my fingers. The corners of her mouth twitch up into a smile. My nipples harden under my hands. I look down to where her breasts are hiding under her robe. It's catching on her own hard nipples, the material clinging to her with static energy. I feel my mouth pooling with saliva as I take her body in – all the times I've looked before were stolen glances; for the first time I have the chance to gaze as longingly as I like.

She uncrosses her legs and her inner thighs are revealed between the split of the robe, loosely tied by its silk cord. I want her to remove it but she doesn't. She continues to watch me as I walk over to my own bed and sit down against my pillows, facing her. My erect nipples press into my palms and, following my own desires, I start to knead my breasts, enjoying the softness. I work my fingers around my nipples, pinching and pulling at the hardness as her gaze tickles at my skin. There is something about her eyes on my naked body that makes me want to perform, to give her a show.

I make myself shiver pleasurably as I trace a line between my breasts, all the way down to my pussy. I see her shoulders lean forwards. She wants to see more.

I don't stop to question my next move; I'm all in now, being led both by what I want and by what I think she wants to see. From my bedside table I retrieve a glass dildo and some lube. I hold the toy up in the air to get her approval, adrenalin pumping through me. Her face seems to flash with excitement. She nods and I see her wetting her lips with her tongue. I lean back against the pillows. I squirt some of the lube into my hand. I move my hand down to my pussy slowly, not letting her see what she wants right away. And then I open my legs wide and begin to massage my wet hand over my already wet pussy. I take the dildo and tease it around my lower lips as I rub my clit with my other lubed-up hand. Pleasure radiates throughout my body; it's as if I'm going hot and cold at the same time.

She's staring at my pussy, at the dildo in one hand and my clit under the other. I pause my movements and wait until she looks back at my eyes. As our gaze connects I plunge the dildo inside me. I moan loudly; I wonder if she can hear. I want her to hear. As I move the dildo in and out, the glass rocking on my G-spot, the fullness completes me. Her eyes have dropped back to my pussy, fixated on it, her mouth opening slightly. I have an urge to put my nipple in her mouth; the fact I can't makes me moan even louder. My pleasure builds and builds. And now I want more from her.

I get up off the bed and walk to the floor-to-ceiling window. I press one of my hands on to the glass and with my other I play with the dildo. She opens her legs wider and the material of her robe falls off her thighs. I can see her pussy and the dark curly bush above it, and I can't look away, my breath caught on my lips. She slips her hand between her legs and touches herself. My heart is beating even faster now she's getting involved. Seeing her there playing too turns me on way more than I thought it would. Lust burns through me and I feel my pussy swelling under my own hands. Her face contorts in pleasure as she moves her fingers over her clit; she started slowly, bringing some of the wetness from her pussy up to rub it, but now she's speeding up. I match her speed with my dildo, pushing and pulling it out fast, making sure the underside of my wrist catches on my clit as I do. She tips her head back as if she's suppressing a moan and the robe falls away from her breasts, exposing them. Jolts of pleasure rise and fall through me as I edge closer and closer to orgasm. But every time I'm close I stop myself; I want to continue watching her. I want us to cum together.

For a brief moment, my eyes wander away from her to scan the area – there are people walking in the street down below minding their own business. A dog walker crouches down to pick up his pooch. I can see a couple having breakfast in another apartment opposite, one feeding the other pancakes in an adorable but sickly way. All these people around who if they glanced up could see either one of us naked and touching ourselves. I'm getting a thrill from the chance more people could look over – that maybe they would join in. The couple could begin to fuck; I'd watch him take her on the kitchen table. Maybe a pedestrian would secretly slip their hand into their trousers.

My eyes flick across to her; her head is rolling back and I can see her fingers dipping in and out of her glistening pussy. She looks really fucking hot and I can tell she's getting closer and closer. I imagine what it would be like if I was there to feel how wet she is, to pinch her hard nipples, if she was rubbing my clit, or better yet swirling her tongue over it. Her chest is heaving and she looks forward again at me, eyes fixing on mine. **As I see her mouth open for a moan to escape, I plunge my dildo in one final time and massage it on my G-spot, slowly moving my hips on it. I lose my focus on her as I fall into a shuddering climax. Pleasure ripples through my body as I let out a loud moan.**

I look up and see her sitting there breathing heavily, looking at me with wide, surprised eyes as if she can't believe that just happened either. I never knew being watched would turn me on so much. We stare at each other while we both catch our breath, still in each other's world. And then she closes her legs, stands and walks out of view of the window. I lose sight of her. But I sit there smiling to myself still. What the hell just happened?

As I get to my feet, I look down: the couple with the pancakes are staring up at me, smiling open-mouthed.

PLAY WITH TEXTURES AND SENSATIONS

When it comes to pleasure, little things make a big impact. Textures and sensations play a big part in what feels good. Using toys that are made of materials such as glass, metal or crystal, for example, can add a whole layer to your experience. On their own they already have a different feel to them from your fingers – they are slippy, naturally cool and hard.

Also think of different sensations you might enjoy – playing with different temperatures, for example, can be an incredibly sensual experience. If you have a non-electric toy, such as a glass dildo, you could put it in the fridge or in a bowl of cold water for a few minutes and experiment with a cold sensation on your sensitive areas. In contrast, you could warm it up in a bowl of warm water to create a heated experience.

As well as using toys you could play with ice, massaging cubes over your body. (For the record, I do not recommend putting an ice cube on someone's cock; I have tried this and it's safe to say I gave him dick freeze.) If you're into more heated play, you can buy body-safe candles and drip wax over your body. As you settle down for some solo sex with the next story now, why not give it a go?

NOTE: It goes without saying that you should use your common sense with this one. As above, don't put electric toys in water, don't put chargeable and electric toys in the fridge – and also don't hurt yourself by making things too cold or too hot.

THE MASTER

READING TIME

<7 MINUTES

THE POV CHARACTER IS

DOMINANT

SEXY CHECKLIST

☐ MASTURBATION

■ CLIT PLAY/FINGERING

☐ CUNNILINGUS

☐ BLOW JOB

■ NIPPLE PLAY

■ VAGINAL PENETRATION

■ ANAL/BUTT PLAY

■ SPANKING

■ SEX TOYS

■ CHOKING

■ BDSM

I know why she's come here.

She's here because for her, the sexiest thing in the world is for me to not just strip her of her clothes but also her power. Maybe even her dignity. She wants the tantalising anticipation of not knowing what's coming next when I tie her up, or stand silently behind her with a paddle in my hand or my erection on her ass. She's here because she wants to be dominated.

I think how small she looks compared to the big bed, where she is sitting in a loose T-shirt and jeans, reading through the waiver, biting her nails with nerves or excitement, or maybe both. She signs it and holds it out for me, fidgeting her foot. I cast my eyes over the document. She hasn't crossed off anything. She's open to it all. I fold it up and put it into the tool belt around my hips.

'Tell me your safe words,' I say.

'Amber for warning.' She swallows. 'Red for stop.'

I tower over her on the bed. 'Aren't you forgetting something?' I say coolly.

'*Master*,' she corrects herself quickly.

I tell her to stand up. I circle round her and see her shoulders tense. When I'm behind her, I lean beside her ear and tell her I'm displeased that she's come dressed so casually, that she must never do so again.

'I'm sorry, Master.' She trips over her words. 'I won't do it again.'

I exhale slowly, wondering whether to accept this apology or not. I decide I will, this time.

I move around to face her. Her eyes are lowered, as I've already taught her to do. I tell her to put her hands into the air. I lift her T-shirt over her head. She isn't wearing a bra and I tell her off for this too. This time I do punish her, pinching one nipple and then the other. She presses her lips together from the pain . . . and the pleasure.

I kneel down and undo her jeans: the button and then the zip, and pull the denim down over her ass and thighs until they're at her feet. I press my nose into her panties and breathe in and out on to them so she can feel my hot breath through the material. She trembles a little. I reach into my tool belt for some scissors. I use them to cut one side of her panties, the cool of the blade on her skin making her wince, and then the other side. The material floats softly to the ground. I stand up and survey her nakedness. She loves me looking at her; she'd stand here all day if she could.

It's time for the restraints. I put a cuff on each of her wrists and ankles, and a collar on for good measure. I tell her to get on all fours and she does. I attach a heavy metal chain to the collar and lead her over to the opposite side of the room, where I tell her to stand up, spread her legs and hold her arms out to the sides, so I can clip the rings on her cuffs to the chains on the large wooden cross I keep there. She does as she's told. She's breathing deeply, something I've told her she must do, but I also know it's from frustration. She wants me to touch her.

I go to the wardrobe in the corner and slowly pull out the drawer. The sound of wood drawing on wood makes her go crazy with expectation. I can feel her eyes on me, wondering what item I'm going to choose. I roll anal beads through my hands so she can see, then put them back down again. Not today. I hold up a riding crop, as if inspecting it, and feel her shifting her weight eagerly behind me. But no. I think I'll choose this one: a flogger, with long leather tails dripping from the handle.

I stand before her. She gazes fearfully at the flogger. I drape it across her body slowly, teasing it across her bare nipples and her chest. She squirms as it tickles her and bites her lip. Then I whip it across her stomach, the sound echoing through the room. She moans a little. I keep going, alternating between her stomach and her thighs. She moans again and closes her eyes, tipping her head back against the cross to expose her throat.

I drop the flogger with a thud to the floor and her eyes flash open, wondering what's going to happen next. I'm sure it's because she doesn't want me to release her from the cross. I don't plan to . . . yet. From inside my tool belt I pull a travel-sized bottle of lube. I squeeze some into my free hand, pocket the bottle and rub my hands together so that they squelch and slide together. Her mouth opens involuntarily.

I stand right in front of her and trace my wet fingers over her inner thigh until they get to her pussy. When I brush against her entrance she takes a sharp intake of air. I pinch her labia sharply. 'Deep breaths only,' I tell her.

'Yes, Master,' she says.

I work my wet fingers over her pussy lips to her clit, slowly circling it. Moans fall out of her, her mouth opening again – an invitation. I plunge my fingers inside her wet pussy, enjoying for myself the warm textured walls closing in against them, and she moans again. I pull my fingers out and insert them into her open mouth to silence her. She licks my fingers, enjoying the taste of herself. I love to tease like this – I know she wants me to repeat my actions, which is why I won't do it.

Instead, I take a small butt plug with a diamond base from my tool belt. I let her watch me suck on it and then move my hand down to her pussy, where I rub it over her entrance before moving it to her butthole. Her body opens to it readily and contracts around it. She sighs, full up, begging to be filled up even more.

I release her from her restraints and tell her to get back on all fours. She crawls on her hands and knees beside me as I lead her by her chain to the bed. I tug on the chain to draw her up on to the bed, face down. I fetch my spreader bar, then attach her legs to it so that they're spread wide apart and can't move. She looks magnificent like this; I can see the diamond butt plug inside her and her glistening, wet pussy.

I kneel in the gap created by her spread legs and rub my hand over her ass. I feel her tense, expecting me to spank her. Instead, I use my other hand to take out a small vibrator. As I click it on and the buzzing starts I see her head, face down on the covers, twitch – she's surprised. Good.

I reach under her and put the vibrator on her pussy and immediately smack her hard across the butt cheek. She gasps. I do it again. Her moans are getting longer and longer. I caress her silky skin between each spank, leaving it seconds between each hit so that she doesn't know when it's coming.

Despite her moans, her breathing has remained slow and steady. I'm pleased with her. I don't always allow her the treatment that's coming next. I rest the vibrator on the sheets directly in between her legs so that she can feel it on her pussy. I get up and undress, let her listen to the sounds of me dropping my shirt to the floor, unclipping my tool belt, unzipping my jeans. I release her from the spreader and lean over her, resting my hard cock on her ass.

'You've been very, very good,' I say into her ear. 'And because you've been so very, very good, I think it's time I fuck you.'

She squirms underneath me; these are her magic words.

I flip her over on to her back and attach the chains on the bedstead to the rings on her cuffs so her arms must stay above her head. I plunge my fingers into her pussy once more so I can steal her wetness and then rub it over my hard, erect cock. I lean my weight down on to her, using my hand to tease my cock over her clit. Then with a deep thrust I push myself inside her.

'Look at me,' I command her. She does as I say, pleased to finally be allowed to look into my face. 'Don't look away,' I tell her, penetrating her again. She leans her head into the sheets and closes her eyes with pleasure. I grab her by the chin. 'Look away again and I'll punish you,' I growl. She nods, trying not to smile. Keeping her eyes fixed on mine. I move my hand from her chin to her throat. I don't squeeze, but I hold it there on her neck firmly, letting her know that at any moment I could.

She pulls at the chains that are holding her arms to the bed; I feel her tense around my cock and know that the butt plug is adding to the intensity of her pleasure – she's getting close. I squeeze her throat more firmly so that she has to fight for the deep breaths I've taught her to take. **Rhythmically, I move, plunging in and out, in and out until her orgasm makes her scream.**

I pull my cock out of her and slide up to her head. She wants to revel in her pleasure, but she's not in control here. I push my cock inside her mouth and she obediently runs her tongue over it. I run my hands through her hair as I say, 'Who's your master?' I pull my cock out and saliva dribbles down her chin.

'You are.' She smiles.

I'll fuck her mouth for another five minutes and then we'll go again.

INTERNAL EXPLORATION

Going inside for lots of people means G-spot action, but actually there are so many ways to feel pleasure when you dip into your vagina. If we think back to when we talked about the clitoris 'wishbone' on page 16, you'll remember I said that it runs either side of the vaginal opening. This means we can feel pleasure from shallow insertion as well as deeper. It can be particularly amazing to explore with the head of a glass, metal or silicone dildo and lots of lube! Here are a few things to try when it comes to shallow play:

- Use the head of a toy to rest gently in your vaginal entrance

- Rock the toy back and forth

- Pull the toy gently in and out

- Curl gently upwards on entry

Each of the above can be an amazing way to tease and build up pleasure slowly. If you want additional sensations then use them in combination with clitoral stimulation.

If you do want to touch your G-spot, below is a basic technique to find it with your fingers – though using your own can be pretty tricky so you might prefer using a toy instead. Tilting your hips up and/or using a pillow underneath your lower back can help you find this spot. (Move the pillow around to find your most comfortable position.)

1. I highly recommend getting lube involved for anything internal – coat your fingers with it.

2. Insert your fingers and bend upwards using the 'come hither' motion for the deeper penetration, where you massage the upper or front 'roof' of your vagina. It's a bit of trial and error, but moving your fingers around until you feel something pleasurable is how you will find your G-spot – it usually feels a little rougher in texture than its surroundings.

3. Now that you're inside and have found your pleasure zone, you can try some different techniques:

   a. Walking your fingers across it.

   b. Curling up in 'come hither' and pulling back out gently against the roof.

   c. Placing a hand on your pubic region and pushing down at the same time as you push up from inside. Think of your hands trying to meet each other.

   d. Using your fingers in circular motions like you're tracing the circle of your vaginal canal.

   e. Using two fingers in a V motion and pull in and out.

For all of these, try different rhythms, pressures and placements to explore.

Don't feel defeated if none of this works for you – finding those angles yourself is REALLY hard and personally I rarely find pleasure this way, but plenty of vulva owners do respond to internal stimulation so it's well worth experimenting and seeing what sparks for you.

Using a toy (see page 102) can be a great way to find internal pleasure because most of them are designed to hit the pleasure zone perfectly, and if you like vibrations inside you then it can really get you going. Once you have the toy inside, you can move it up and around to find the area that gives you that tingle. Personally, I like to use the toy in a rocking motion that slightly mimics the 'come hither' motion to enjoy the pleasure most!

Hopefully there's something here that you'd like to give a go in the next story; if you're sure internal exploration isn't for you then pick a different tip to try!

MY DEMON

READING TIME

<10 MINUTES

THE SEXUAL PARTNER IS

FRIGHTENING

SEXY CHECKLIST

☐ MASTURBATION
☐ CLIT PLAY/FINGERING
☐ CUNNILINGUS
☐ BLOW JOB
☐ NIPPLE PLAY
■ VAGINAL PENETRATION
☐ ANAL/BUTT PLAY
☐ SPANKING
☐ SEX TOYS
■ CHOKING
■ BDSM

I can feel his eyes on the back of my neck, again. My skin prickles with a cold sweat.

I'm at a house party, dancing in the living room, the thumping of the bass reverberating through my body. Every time I look over my shoulder he's there ready to catch my eyes. I don't know who he is but he's been watching me all night.

I shudder and take myself out of the room to get another drink and to find some respite from him. In the kitchen, I look over the mess of bottles and cups to find vodka and a suitable mixer, grab and pour. I've made it too strong; it stings my throat as I gulp it down. When I look up, I half expect to see the stranger standing in front of me, but the kitchen is empty. I should be relieved. A group of people bustle past talking loudly and laughing; they stagger into the garden. I should join them but I'm too lost in thought. Was I slightly disappointed he wasn't there? I bat the thought away; of course not, he's got massive stalker vibes.

I walk back into the living room, fresh drink in hand. I look around the room at the bobbing heads and churning bodies; he's nowhere to be seen. My stomach sinks a little. I'm feeling the absence of his attention. But I'm relieved too, right? I think so. I slip back into the trance of the music, moving my body, seducing the room.

And that's when I hear it, like a whisper in my ear.

'Leave.'

A chill coats my skin. I look around me, my eyes widening in shock. Was that real or am I just drunk? I don't think I've had that much to drink, but hearing voices is a clear sign I should stop. I can feel my heart beating against my ribcage, hard and fast. I look around at my friends – they're dancing obliviously, swaying their hips and grinding on the air.

'Leave now.'

Goosebumps rise all over my arms, my heart thudding as loud as the bass in the room. What the fuck is happening to me? My eyes dart around the room looking for a reason, something to clarify what I'm hearing.

That's when I see him. He's waiting in the doorway; I catch his eye for a split second and I swear his eyes flash amber, like a flickering flame. He turns and walks away, towards the kitchen and the back door.

'Follow.' The voice tickles the inside of my ears. I feel curiosity building inside me, almost like an invisible force pulling at me to walk out of the room, to leave the house, to follow him. So I do.

The bright lights of the kitchen seem to sting me as I go to the door. The darkness of the garden feels more alluring suddenly. I spot a flash of amber in the start of the forest-line fifty feet away. He's leading me into the depth of the trees. I open the door and step out into the cold air of the night, gasping at the chill wiping over my skin. A question circles non-stop around my mind as the damp grass licks my bare feet: who is he? *What* is he?

As I reach the trees, I look back. The thumping of the bass in the house is being replaced by the snap of the twigs under my steps. With no shoes on, they bite into my soles. My skin prickles in the cool air, my dress not covering enough skin to keep me warm. As I move further into the thicket, I feel very alone, the darkness surrounding me, the house no longer visible.

The wind howls in a feral sort of way, and it is as if the air around me trembles. There is something here with me. I whip my head around, searching for it.

Suddenly I can't breathe. An ice-cold grip tightens around my throat from behind me – I splutter, moving my hands to my neck, clawing at whatever invisible force has hold of me.

'You're all alone.' A soft seductive voice brushes my right ear. 'Nowhere to run,' I hear now in my left ear. 'Nowhere to hide.' His grip momentarily loosens and I gasp for air. My mind races. I'm going to die; I'm going to die right here in this forest. Why did I follow him? What spell has he cast on me?'

'I've been watching you,' the voice says, his grip tightening again. 'You are fascinating to me. The way your body moves. Your skin in the light. Your hair, your eyes. You're not like the other humans.' My pulse is throbbing under his grip, my mouth parted, needing air.

In a split second I am released and alone again. I double over, spluttering, clutching at my throat, the cold air piercing my lungs as they refill. My heart is the only thing I can hear, thudding dramatically.

'I want you.' This time the voice is inside my head, like it was in the house. 'Will you be mine?'

'What are you? What do you want from me?' My voice is rough and panicked.

Suddenly he's there, standing in front of me. The darkness of the forest makes him impossible to make out apart from his eyes alight like the flames of a roaring fire. A smile curls from the corners of his mouth, revealing a full set of spiked teeth that glint in the moonlight.

'I want you to be mine,' he says. Before I can blink he's pushed me up against the nearest tree. The bark is cutting into my back. I look up into his fiery eyes. His cool breath teases over my lips, sending a flutter of anticipation down my throat and between my legs. His form has changed from the man I saw at the party. Claws instead of nails. Skin not a colour I know how to describe. He towers over me.

I close my eyes tightly, pressing my hands into the tree behind me, telling myself I'm in a nightmare.

Suddenly: my heartbeat slows down. I feel . . . calm, comforted. I don't feel threatened any more, I feel . . . turned on. I open my eyes. This beautiful creature wants me. He touches his finger to my lips. My skin fizzes from the contact.

'I know what you want,' he says, his voice melting the inside of my mind. There's a tickling sensation behind my eyes. 'I know all your deepest, darkest desires.' His lips curl into a fierce grin and his eyes flash darker. He leans into me and kisses my open mouth. It's like no other kiss I've ever experienced. I shiver at the feel of his cold lips against mine, but his tongue is hot and feels almost electric. His saliva is sweet as it rushes into my mouth and trickles down my throat. Now we've started, I kiss him back hungrily: I want more.

He pulls me forward and spins me around to push my face on to the trunk of the tree. His body leans into my back. Something hard presses against my bum. It feels . . . big.

I know what I want to happen next. Without me doing anything, without him touching me, my knickers start to slide down my legs to the dirt. He pulls up my dress to reveal my ass, taking his hand to massage the softness. I feel something wet dripping over the back of me, the saliva dripping from his mouth, wetting me ready for him. The wetness feels cool as it disappears between my ass cheeks and to my entrance, my pussy engorged. I feel his hardness press between my cheeks; it feels different to the cocks I have had before. Cold and hard, but somehow with a fire at the core. I want to turn around to look at it, but just as I try, he pushes my head into the tree, keeping me in place.

He starts to rub the head of his cock in-between my legs, teasing my entrance. Ripples of anticipatory pleasure unfurl from my opening, and the rub of his hard end sends unexpected but not unwelcome pain as I stretch to take him in. I gasp at the shock. He growls, that feral growl I heard on the wind before, as he plunges the rest of his enormous cock inside me. I inhale sharply as he slips inside so easily for something so big. He thrusts hard and deep, which makes me let out a whimper of pleasure. If his tongue is electric, then so is his cock. Vibrations surge through me, causing a sensation of pure euphoria. He grabs my hair and pulls my head to the side as he licks up my neck. More electric shocks, his saliva crackling as it touches my skin.

Every touch, movement, breath sends waves of pleasure though my body as he fiercely fucks me from behind, panting and growling like an animal. Forced to take him inside me as he pins me to the tree, I am uncontrollably wet around his cock, feeling it dripping down my legs. His hands claw at my back, cutting my skin; I can feel my warm blood beginning to run. He leans into me, licking at the wounds; it stings as he touches me. It hurts so good. My adrenalin pumps with the anticipation of the pain, and yet somehow it feels comforting at the same time because he's tending to me. I feel myself falling into another world of pleasure, an *underworld* of pleasure.

'I'm going to finish inside you,' he whispers into my ear. 'I'm going to make you mine.' His words make me moan loudly. I want him to cum inside me, I want him to fill me up, I want him to own me. And he knows.

He thrusts deeper and harder, moving fiercely and forcefully. I can feel him growing inside me, bigger and bigger, the vibrations making me hum from the inside as he stretches me. It turns into pulsing – as if his cock is pulsing the beat of the bass I was dancing to earlier. **Suddenly I feel a warmness inside me that takes my breath away and the pleasure starts rocketing through my body like a fire catching alight. Spasms ricochet through me as I reach the peak of my pleasure. This orgasm is like nothing I've felt before, as his cock engorges to fill the curves of my insides.** My legs buckle as he holds me close to him.

He hugs me into his body, keeping his cock inside me.

'You're mine.' I'm his. He kisses me all over my back, kneading my body, nursing me.

I want to turn around and kiss him, but as soon as the thought enters my mind, he's gone. The weight of his body no longer supports me, my legs buckle and I fall to my knees. I sit there, speechless. I look down at my open legs. A blue liquid is dripping out of me. I put a finger to it and take it to my mouth. It sparks and tastes like pleasure itself.

I sit in the dark forest all alone, unmoving, not sure what to do with myself. I am his. But will I see him again?

TIP 13:

NIPPLES!

Our bodies have so many different erogenous zones, and one of my favourites to play with is nipples as they hold lots of nerve endings and love to get some attention. Like the clit, we all have varying sensitivity levels here, so it's really about experimenting and finding what feels good for you. I hope you'll give it a go throughout the next story.

So how do we touch them? You might want to try over fabric first to figure out your sensitivity levels. Try rubbing around the nipple in circular motions. Pinching and pulling the nipples. Massaging or rubbing them with a bigger surface area like your palm.

If you really enjoy these sensations on your nipples you might want to invest in some toys like nipple clamps or suckers. Clamps squeeze on to your nipples feeling like a big pinch – it's painful but sometimes pain heightens pleasure in a big way. For your first time using clamps, I would recommend buying some that you can monitor the tightness with, so you can start off soft and build up to find out what you enjoy. Suckers are a little different because they work with air compression: you squeeze them on to your nipple and the air vacuum attaches them. Again, you can work with pressure and the tightness of the sucker.

One of my favourite things to do during solo sex with my nipples is use a clit suction toy. Set it to the intensity that you like and then place the sucker over your nipple or move it around the areola. It literally feels like someone is sucking on your nipple! This can work really well with lube to get that extra-real feel of a mouth.

FIRST TIME
WITH A GIRL

READING TIME

<7 MINUTES

THE SEXUAL PARTNER IS

CONFIDENT

SEXY CHECKLIST

☐ MASTURBATION
■ CLIT PLAY/FINGERING
■ CUNNILINGUS
☐ BLOW JOB
■ NIPPLE PLAY
☐ VAGINAL PENETRATION
☐ ANAL/BUTT PLAY
☐ SPANKING
☐ SEX TOYS
☐ CHOKING
☐ BDSM

My friend Elba is beautiful, I think to myself. I take a sip of wine; it slips down easily, making me feel warm from the inside out. We're in my living room, sitting close to each other on a sofa with cushions you can sink into, the curtains drawn against a stormy night where the trees are doing backbends in the wind. She's telling me the ins and outs of her break-up with her girlfriend. While she talks I notice how much I like the way her hair is falling past her shoulders, how smooth and glowing her skin looks in the lamplight, how round her cheeks are, how her eyes always glint a little mischievously. And her lips. Her lips are like the sofa cushions – I could sink into them.

This is all news to me. I've known Elba for years and I've never thought this about her before – or about any other woman. Yes, I've often thought how beautiful women are, how soft and elegant they can be, but it hadn't occurred to me that it might mean something more. Tonight, my pussy's telling me it does. It feels hot and alive in my knickers, as if it's swelling against the material. I'm sure Elba knows I'm looking at her like this – she keeps touching her chest and her neck, leading my eyes there.

'What about you?' She suddenly changes the topic, playing with the rim of her wine glass. 'Are you dating anyone?'

Normally that would be a friendly enquiry, not a leading question, but tonight . . . there's an energy in the air.

'No,' I say. Hoping she'll pick up on the intention, I test the water by saying, 'I've had enough recently; men aren't doing it for me at all.'

She pauses, looking directly at me as she contemplates my response. Does she know what I want yet? Then she says, 'That's good to know.'

She moves her bare leg against mine. A static travels through me as her knee slips by my thigh. She doesn't move it away. My pussy quivers.

'Why?' I ask hopefully, feeling like a teenager, flirting for the first time again.

She doesn't say anything in response; instead, she leans very slowly towards me, giving me the time and space to pull back if I want to. I don't. Her lips land on mine. They're softer than I ever thought lips could be; they melt into my own like Vaseline.

'I didn't know you liked girls,' she breathes, an inch from my face.

'I didn't know either,' I admit.

She puts a hand on the side of my face. 'Do you want this?'

I bite my lip. 'Yes,' I breathe. 'But I've never been with a woman before; I don't know what to do.'

'That's what they all say,' she giggles.

Now I'm pulling open the door into my moonlit bedroom. Behind me, she places her hands on my waist and I feel her pressed up against my back – the softness of her boobs, belly and thighs. She spins me around and kisses me. This time her tongue's in my mouth and I love how wet it feels in there. It feels different to kissing a man, it feels doughy, sensual; it feels liberating. I put my hands in her hair and run them over her neck.

'What do you want?' she says into my ear, then sucks on my earlobe.

I don't know where the confidence comes from but I say, 'I want to see *you*.'

I feel her lips curl up into a grin by my ear, her cheek pressing against mine.

She steps back and takes off her top. She isn't wearing a bra and in the dim light her breasts bounce lightly as they fall out. I feel my nipples tighten as they become erect inside the soft cotton shell of my bra. Inside my pussy, my pulse strengthens. She takes both my hands and moves them up her torso to rest on her breasts. I've never touched anybody's but my own before. I squeeze them gently – hers feel so different to mine. They are full and heavy against my palms. Her nipples feel like velvet and they harden pleasingly against my fingertips as I caress them. A small moan escapes her lips.

I'm impatient to see more. I move my hands down and undo the button on her shorts, pull down the zip, tug at the material so that they drop over her bare thighs and hit the carpeted floor.

'Now you,' she says.

I undress and love the feel of her eyes on me as I do. I go one step further than her and pull down my knickers. She eats me up with her gaze.

'You're beautiful,' she says.

She slides down her own knickers and then takes me by the hand and leads me to the bed. The duvet moulds to my body, softly caressing my bare skin.

She goes straight for my breasts, her warm breath tickles my skin. She wraps her lips over my nipple. The suction feels comforting and arousing at the same time, heat rippling through me. I close my eyes and breathe deeply, noticing the feel of her soft hands as they explore my stomach and breasts. This unknown sexual territory has heightened all my senses. The ache inside my pussy is mounting and I unconsciously rock my hips towards her to get her attention. She notices and responds accordingly, running her hand down my stomach until she reaches my pussy. She plunges two fingers in, releasing some of my tension, but teasingly doesn't move them, still concentrating on my nipples with her lips instead. I let out a moan of pleasure and frustration. She giggles, knowing what I want.

'My turn,' she says, slipping out her fingers. I don't want her to stop, I want her tongue inside my pussy, but I'm too excited to explore her body. I move down the bed so that I can sit between her legs. I don't look at her pussy just yet – instead, I trace her whole body with both my hands, squeezing her breasts, stroking her waist, bending her legs at the knee so I can stroke the smooth underside of her thigh. I can't believe how natural this all feels.

Then I look at her pussy. I've never seen one so closely before; even in the darkness I can see enough to know I want to taste it. Her petal-like labia blush with arousal; above, her clit is hidden by delicate folds of skin. I bend down towards it, then hesitate, not knowing how to start.

'Circle my clit with your tongue,' she says. I follow her guidance; her skin tastes sweet and salty. As I orbit she lets out a moan of pleasure. The intensity of tonight must be as hot for her as it is for me.

'Now suck on it.' I do as she says. I love having my mouth on her and she pushes up against me appreciatively, her hands reaching down and gripping my hair, pulling me close. I feel her tense and tighten as my rhythm intensifies. But this pleasure is as much mine as it is hers and I want more of her. I can't wait to know what she feels like – my fingers slip over the folds of her and I push two fingers inside her pussy. It's warmer and wetter than I'd imagined. Hearing her moans drive me to push further inside her, pulling up at her G-spot, my tongue still on her clit. She's tensing around my fingers, pushing against my mouth – but before she cums, she pulls me up to her level.

She slips her thigh between my legs and presses rhythmically on me. We're tangled together, thrusting our thighs against each other's pussies. Her movements rub directly on my clit as I mirror her actions and because we're both already so close to cumming, heat starts to crash through me as we lock into a kiss. **Our bodies mould together, pulsing, rocking, thrusting into one, and our breath is feverish on each other's necks.**

I cum first, and then she does – body on body, mouth on mouth.
Wow, I mouth the word into her shoulder but nothing comes out.
'How was that?' she asks me.
'That was like nothing else . . . ' I'm still trying to catch my breath.
'So you like girls, huh?' She smiles, her beautiful lips curling. We both giggle. I hold on to her, so happy that I've tried something new.

TIP 14:

SELF-MASSAGE

Throughout the next story may I suggest you get sensual with yourself by using some vagina-safe massage oils? Little tip here: it's best to use oil-based lubes.

Who doesn't love a massage? We often forget that we can touch ourselves in these ways, so here's a self-massage to try:

1. Set the mood (relaxing music, candles, heating on – whatever feels right for you) and get yourself naked. Lay down a towel if you're worried about getting messy!

2. Take a small dollop of oil and spread it across your hands and fingers. If your hands are cold, you might want to warm them up – equally you might quite like the cold sensation!

3. Gently massage the oil into your inner thighs and tease close to your vulva. (You can take more time with the tease if you like, for example working from your feet and ankles, all the way up your calves to your thighs.)

4. Before diving into your vulva, tease and massage your breasts and nipples if this is something you enjoy.

5. Massage from your inner thighs to your outer labia. This part is all about building the tension and heat to the max before diving into the main pleasure zones.

6. When you're ready, massage around your clit and over your inner labia. Take your time to explore what sensations feel good. You might want to look at pages 84 and 76 for ideas on how to directly and indirectly touch your clit.

7. Relax, keep going and enjoy. The aim isn't to orgasm, but if you do that's an amazing bonus!

MY HAPPY ENDING

READING TIME
<10 MINUTES

THE SEXUAL PARTNER IS
KIND

SEXY CHECKLIST
☐ MASTURBATION
■ CLIT PLAY/FINGERING
■ CUNNILINGUS
☐ BLOW JOB
☐ NIPPLE PLAY
☐ VAGINAL PENETRATION
☐ ANAL/BUTT PLAY
☐ SPANKING
☐ SEX TOYS
☐ CHOKING
☐ BDSM

A twist of my key satisfyingly releases the front-door lock, and I haul myself over the threshold, and drop my bag with a clatter, exhaustedly kicking my shoes off on to the wooden floor. My bare feet feel sore on the hard surface as I walk to the living room; the muscles across my back are taut as I melt on to the sofa. I reach down to my feet and start kneading the week's tension out of them with my thumbs – it feels so good to be touched, to feel the nerves in my toes respond to the silky surface of my hands. Although it would be better if someone else was here to do it for me. It's been a long time since anyone has touched me like that . . .

On the coffee table in front of me is a massage voucher my friend Diana bought me for my birthday a few days ago; I've been so busy I haven't had a chance to do any celebrating yet. On the spur of the moment I dial the number on the voucher, feeling half-asleep until—

'Good evening.' His voice is soft, sensual, it almost purrs. 'Masseur at your service – what can I do for you?'

'Hello!' I find myself saying eagerly, far more alert than when I picked up the phone. 'I'd love to book a massage. I don't suppose you have any availability right now, do you? I know it's late notice but I've had a long week and I have a birthday voucher . . . '

'Your birthday, you say?' His tongue rolls over the 'r's like the soft rumbles of thunder. I hold my breath hopefully. 'Well, in that case of course I have the availability.'

We exchange details and as I put the phone down, butterflies flurry through my stomach. What does a man with a voice as seductive as that look like? I wonder.

Half an hour later, a buzz at the doorbell notifies me that the wait to find out is over. I check myself in the mirror before opening the door. Too busy thinking about my own appearance, my jaw drops unintentionally. There, standing just feet away from me, is a man who looks as if he's stepped out of a shampoo commercial. His hair looks so beautifully wavy and soft. I have an involuntary daydream of running my hand through it. He gives me a knowing grin as I force myself to close my mouth.

'I'm your birthday present,' he says.

A smile tugs at the corners of my lips. I make a mental note to thank Diana profusely with many bottles of wine.

He sets up the massage table in my living room and as he walks past me I catch the smell of him – mint shower gel, clean and fresh. I find I'm mesmerised by the fluid movements of his bare arms below a bright white T-shirt. The muscles along his forearms tense pleasingly – I realise I'm twirling my hair like a schoolgirl.

'I'm ready for you.'

My eyes linger on his body as he gestures me to the massage table. His hands look strong and somehow tender at the same time. An inappropriate hunger courses through me.

'I'll step out while you get undressed. Just hop under the sheet and I'll be back in a moment.'

I take off my clothes, fold everything and place them on the sofa. It feels liberating to be standing in my living room naked. I make a note to myself to do this more often. I wonder if he ever peeks as people get undressed. The thought of him doing it now tingles the hairs on my arms.

I slip myself under the sheet on the massage table and settle my face into the small cosy hole.

There's a faint knock on the living-room door, then light footsteps slowly pad across the floor, gently getting louder. I see his bare feet down in front of me. He doesn't utter a word before pulling the sheet down. The cloth tickles my skin as he drapes it over the small of my back, my bum dangerously close to exposure. Heat rises in my face, blushing excitedly at what his eyes are laying on. Instinctively I close my eyes; every sound is heightened now. I can hear my breath and the click of a bottle opening, one of my favourite ASMR sounds, a squeeze of liquid into his palm, the slick rubbing of his hands as he warms up the oil. I tense, and then—

His hands gently touch my skin for the first time, right at the top of my back, near my neck. It sends little shockwaves through my body; my stomach flutters as if I've just dropped down a roller-coaster track. But as the strokes and the pressure increase, I relax into it. I notice that his hands are the perfect temperature, warm, as if they could melt into me.

He moves his hands down to the curves of my shoulder blades, interspersing firm strokes with soft tickles that feel . . . sexual in intent – but that's just my imagination, right?

Further down his hands stroke, until they are nestled around my waist. I bite my lip and let out a little moan without realising.

'Does that feel good?' His voice is so intimate, as if he's whispering into my ear.

I feel a rush of heat tingle in my cheeks again. I stop myself from gushing and opt for: 'Very nice, thanks.'

He laughs; it's a soft, kind, assured laugh. 'Don't be shy about saying what you like. If it feels good, then you should say it feels good.'

I press my lips together with a sharp inhale. That was *definitely* sexual, wasn't it? For some inexplicable reason I give him a thumbs-up. I don't know how but I can feel him grinning to himself. He catches my hand by the wrist and gently places it back on the table;
I wonder if he can feel my embarrassment – or my pulse quickening.

I fall back into a trance as his warm, slippery hands glide over me. He's made it down to the small of my back, where he works his palms into the juicy muscles I have at the top of my bum. He pauses his hands, his flat palms half resting on my skin, half resting on my bum covered up with the sheet. My eyes flutter open, my heartbeat suddenly drumming. 'If you like,' he says, 'I can give you a proper glute massage?'

My eyes widen with his suggestion – is this really happening? I flick my hand up again with a thumbs-up. This time he takes my hand in his as he gently places it down again.

'Your wish is my command,' he breathes, and pulls the sheet down to just above my knees. The rippling of the fabric sends a breeze of cool air up my spine, a wild contrast to the heat of his gaze as his eyes roam over my bare cheeks. Just before I start to get nervous about agreeing to this, his hands touch me. They work into my bum, kneading its squishy tissues and muscles. The touch sends a heat into my loins and my pussy flutters achingly with the attention my body is receiving. It feels so, so good, and I let out a moan. The tenderness of his touch, the firm but gentle pressure, feels completely and utterly pleasurable. I can feel myself swelling between my legs, wanting his attention to move down. I notice his breathing is becoming deep and slow above me, which I start to mimic unintentionally.

I'm desperate for him to move his hands to where I want them. 'It feels good,' I say, encouragingly.

'Yes?'

'*Really* good.'

As if I've said the magic words, his fingers work their way around the very top of my thighs, reaching in and around, pulling at my flesh. He's so close to causing me ridiculous amounts of pleasure, it's almost as if he's teasing me on purpose. My mind swirls into pools of desires, thoughts of him going just that little bit further, plunging himself into my already lubed-up entrance. Moans of pleasure are escaping my mouth in an uncontainable way and I don't care any more. He knows what he's doing.

And just when I think I might explode from the suspense, his hands pull my legs apart, he spreads my butt and I feel something completely different. Something wet and hot moves over my naked pussy, warm breath tickling my clit. His lips are on my vulva lips, his tongue working into my folds. His hands are still working on me, kneading my butt, getting closer and closer, spreading me out so he can see all of me. My head is in the clouds, my eyes tightly shut, I feel like I'm dreaming. Is this actually happening?

Then his expert fingers plunge inside me; they rock on my special spot, stroking me gently but firmly from the inside. An internal massage like I've never felt before. I gasp in pleasure, my hands wrap around the sheet underneath me, holding on for my life as he fully removes every inch of stress that was in my body. His warm tongue is wrapping around my clit, encircling it; his fingers glide in and out of me, in and out. The air in the room feels like it's wrapping me up in a warm blanket. Static tingles radiate all over my body, spreading the sensations deep inside my pussy. I think . . . I'm going to . . .

Like lightning striking, I feel a pleasure within that makes me convulse, spasming around him. His tongue spiralling around me, fingers penetrating deeply. A rush of energy soars through me as I let out one final moan, releasing the last of the tension that I had previously been feeling.

I wake up on my sofa, my eyes adjusting to the street-lamp light coming through the curtains. The room is quiet and still. My body feels like jelly in the best way possible, not an ache in reach. I look around . . . what just happened?

I see a small piece of paper on my coffee table in my direct eyeline. I grab it and read:

You fell asleep during your massage. Didn't want to disturb the Sleeping Beauty. Until next time x

TIP 15:

POSITIONS

If you're like me, you might find yourself repeating the same thing again and again when you masturbate, without switching things up to find out if there are different ways to find your pleasure. It's so easy to get a little lazy when it comes to solo sex, but that's why we're here, right?

Getting in a routine and habit can lead to our brains linking a position to a certain type of pleasure, orgasm or experience. We can then find ourselves struggling to enjoy other positions and situations because there's a possibility of disappointment or dissatisfaction. This is why it's so worth mixing things up and exploring different avenues of feeling pleasure without putting pressure on ourselves – especially as it can also inspire new things to try in your external sex life. But equally, trying out a new position might bring way more pleasure than you ever thought possible!

Remember that orgasm doesn't need to be your goal – you could give a new position a go just to see what the experience is like and to assess how much pleasure it gives you.

Here are some positions you might want to try masturbating in:

- On your knees with your heels beneath your bum. This creates great access to the front and the back.

- On your back, with a pillow under your hips to prop up your pelvis. Great for finding that pleasure zone within.

- On all fours – using one hand to touch yourself.

- Standing up, with one leg raised up on an object such as a bed or chair.

- On your belly with your hand or vibrator between your legs.

As well as trying out different positions you might want to switch up your location. Perhaps on the sofa, or maybe in the bath or shower – download the audiobook and you can listen while you play! PS: If you find a new position that feels incredible, please slide into my DMs because I need to know about it.

THE SHERIFF AND THE BANDIT

READING TIME
>10 MINUTES

THE SEXUAL PARTNER IS
OBEDIENT

SEXY CHECKLIST
☐ MASTURBATION
■ CLIT PLAY/FINGERING
■ CUNNILINGUS
■ BLOW JOB
☐ NIPPLE PLAY
■ VAGINAL PENETRATION
☐ ANAL/BUTT PLAY
☐ SPANKING
☐ SEX TOYS
☐ CHOKING
■ BDSM

The swing doors swoosh back and forth after I enter the saloon, the breeze it creates sweeping my hair forwards. The smell of liquor and sweaty men hits me like a punch in the face – but it's a smell you get used to when you're one of the West's only female bandits.

I'm new to town but this looks as good a bar as any. There's someone playing a tune on the piano, my face isn't staring back at me from a WANTED poster, and no one's told me to get out – not all of the bars out here let women into their fine establishments. Not that I ever let a small thing like rules stop me.

I walk over to a barstool with my name on it, taking my pride and joy – my leather bull-hide hat – off my head as I do so and placing it on the countertop. I order a whisky, straight up, from the barkeep, then swing around on my stool, laying my arms back on the bar to get a good view of my surroundings. My eyes are caught by something glinting in the back pocket of a dusty old man sitting with his back towards me. Something gold. Too good to pass up.

I spare a look around: everyone's laughing or drunkenly hanging over their tables. I stroll towards the piano, whisky in hand, under the pretence of looking at what music sheets are on the top. On my way back, I lean down and swipe myself the gold watch.

I'll be out of here now, just as soon as I've got my hat. As I fit it on my head, I glance down at the gold watch laying heavily in my palm. Nice haul.

And then my wrist is caught by a firm, large hand.

'Miss, I don't believe that is yours,' a velvety voice close to my ear says.

Before I look up to see the man's face, I see what's pinned to his chest: a shiny star. The town's local sheriff. Motherfucker.

I'm a cat, my mother used to say; I can always land on my feet. And I can see from the way the sheriff's Adam's apple is almost nervously bobbing as he swallows and the way his grip on my wrist is solid but not rough, that the best way to land on my feet this time is to bat my eyelashes at him.

'Sheriff, ain't I lucky to have bumped into you?' I say theatrically. 'I just found this on the floor over there and was looking for a strong, law-abiding man to hand it in to.'

I remove his hand from my wrist, turn it over so it's palm up and place the gold watch into it, closing his fingers for him and giving them a stroke for good measure. I look up into his eyes to see if it's done the trick. I'll admit I'm caught off-guard. His eyes are a handsome light brown, a little reddy in the oil lamplight, like good leather.

Letting him see my face, it turns out, was the wrong thing to do. 'I thought I recognised you,' he says shrewdly, narrowing those good-looking brown eyes. With the hand not holding the watch, he pulls out a WANTED poster and slams it on the countertop. Whoever drew my face has a real talent.

I try to tell him I can explain but he's already got the handcuffs out and is pinning me to the bar, my hands behind my back. I struggle against him but it's pointless, those big hands belong to strong arms, and before I know it, he's yanking me towards the swing doors and marching me across the street to the jail, our way lit by the bright moon above.

I've been in worse cells, I think, as he throws me in the only one – no snoring drunk man in here. I wait for the sheriff to tell me that it's late and he'll deal with me tomorrow, so I can start thinking of my grand escape plan. But he lights up a lamp, plonks himself down on a chair right next to the cell bars and puts his hat over his face as if he's ready to go to sleep.

'No little lady to run home to?' I suggest.

'You've got a reputation, miss – no way am I giving you a chance to break out. I'm not letting you out of my sight.'

'You'll need to take your hat off then,' I joke weakly.

His hat's only covering his eyes. I can see his mouth from underneath it and it upturns in a smile. A good-looking smile to go with his good-looking eyes.

I lean against the wooden wall, my hands still trapped behind my back, and wonder if this one might be beyond even me. Then I have an idea.

It's a cold night and in the opposite corner of the small jail is a blanket. Shivering for good measure, I ask the sheriff if he'd be so kind as to let me have it. He looks suspiciously at me, but moves to get it all the same. Good-looking eyes, good-looking smile, and now a good-looking ass. *Stop checking him out and concentrate*, I think to myself.

He holds out the blanket to me through the bars. I turn around to remind him of my handcuffed hands. 'You'll have to wrap it around me,' I say.

He doesn't protest – he likes being near me, I'm certain of it. I stay with my back to him as he unlocks the cell door, so he can put the blanket easily over my shoulders. Luckily my hands are in the ideal position. When he's close enough to me, I run my hands over his groin. I can feel the swell of his cock under his jeans. He pauses for a second then puts his hand on my shoulder and roughly spins me round. He's trying to look angry but his reddish-brown eyes are wanting. I've got him.

I don't have the patience to wait for him to decide what happens next, so in true bandit style I make the first move. My lips press into his warm mouth and I slip my tongue into his – he tastes like smoke and whisky. He pushes me off him.

'There's no use pretending you don't want to,' I say quietly. I lick my lips. 'If you undo my handcuffs, in return it can all be yours.' Slowly I turn away from him once more so he's facing my trapped hands. I wait. Five. Four. Three. Two—

He's at my back. I can feel him breathing on my neck, his fingers graze my skin as he unlocks the handcuffs. I turn back around. I look towards the door of the cell. The smart thing to do would be to dash out right now, slam the door shut and disappear into the night. But those eyes, those eyes are looking at me with more lust than all the customers at the town brothel put together.

I run my hands over the stubble on his jaw and then I kiss him again. It's as if I've set the cannon off – our faces are suddenly locked together and his hands move almost frantically over me, searching my body. I start unbuttoning his shirt and he mirrors my actions but can't quite grasp my belts and buckles. I think it's time I took control of this sheriff.

I push him away with a force that knocks him back a few steps. He looks bewildered and horny all at once.

'Undress,' I order him.

There's that smile again. He starts to grapple with his own clothing. His boots, then his belt, tugging at the leather to release it slowly from the denim loops. It drops to the floor with a loud thud. My mouth is moist as I watch him step out of his jeans. Each item of his clothing lands heavily on the wooden floor as he takes it off. Until there he is, standing completely naked in front of me: his hard cock saluting me. He stands watching me, waiting.

I undress too, unlatching my various belts – one for my guns, another for my chaps. He watches me as if he's never seen a woman's naked body before. His gaze combined with the cool of the night air on my body is making all my sensations extra alert. My nipples twinge as they harden; my pussy feels hot down below.

I decide to take the law into my own hands. I bend down and pick up the belt he dropped. Then I pull him roughly by the arm to the bars, force his wrists to sit together against one of the long poles and use the belt to tie him into position. His silence and the continued presence of his erection confirms to me that he has no objections, though he says, 'This wasn't exactly what I had in mind, miss.'

I smile at him. 'I didn't say you could talk.'

I leave the cell – a flicker of fear runs across his face but I'm not going anywhere yet. I move around to face him on the other side of the bars. I look down between his legs. A gem of his liquid excitement slowly forms on the helmet of his cock, glinting in the light. I run my hand down his body as I get to my knees, then take him in my mouth. At my first touch he lets out a sharp, excited exhale. I tease his shaft with my lips and tongue, using a hand to hold it firmly within my control. My saliva drips down him as I move rhythmically up and down it. I look up at him and seeing my eyes seems to give him all the more pleasure. His moans excite me and spur me on – but he needs to know tonight isn't just about him and his pleasure, it's my turn now.

'Get on your knees,' I tell him as I wipe my mouth. He does as I say, sliding his wrists and the belt that's connecting them to the bar down as he goes. I take the chair he was sitting on before, sit down and use the bars to pull myself forward so that I'm flush with them. Then I spread my legs, pussy perfectly positioned in one of the gaps. His eyes are transfixed on it: hot, wet and ready for him. I feel a drip travelling down my inner thigh which I catch with a finger. He watches me as I take my finger with my own wetness and slowly trace my tongue over it.

'Lick it,' I say.

I feel him breathe out a heavy wanting breath as his tongue moves over my pussy, finding its way over my labia to my clit. A rush of heat moves through my body, it feels like I'm being lapped on by flames. I look around me for something to grip onto as the pleasure builds: first the bars, then his hair, then I claw my nails into his shoulder, which causes him to move faster and further into me. Moans of pleasure release from the depths of my throat, purring like a tiger released from her cage. He moans too, the vibrations only adding to the hot sensations rippling through me.

It's too much, I need more.

I scrape the chair back, see the disappointment crest his face as I close my legs and get up – but he ain't seen it all yet. I go back into the cell and stand behind him, my wet, dripping pussy pressed against his back as I untie the belt. The taste of freedom turns him on and he twists around on his knees, ready to put his hands on me. I give him a playful slap, 'No touching,' and he obediently drops them. 'Lie down with your hands above your head.'

He does as he's told and I belt his wrists back on the bar again. Seeing his body laid out for me like a banquet is something else. His thick thighs, his tensing stomach, his rock-hard cock, standing to attention, ready for me. I stand with a leg either side of his groin and look down at his reddish-brown eyes as he surveys the whole of my body above him. I've never seen so much desire in a man before.

'Who's in charge here, Sheriff?'

He swallows. 'You are, miss.'

'Good boy.' And with that I crouch down, lowering myself on to him, on to all of him. He slips inside me, slowly filling me up completely. My pussy grabs on to every inch of his cock, pulling him deeper inside me. His eyes roll back into his head briefly before he targets them back on to mine. I grab his neck to steady me as I start to rock back and forth. He's hitting all the right places, the head of his cock rubbing on that spot inside that feels real good. I can feel the heat building, pleasure surging through my whole body.

I abruptly stop and stand off his cock. Anger flashes across his eyes as he frowns, a frustrated groan escaping his lips. But he's a good boy who already knows better than to say anything. I turn around so my back is to him and sit back down on his cock. The angle against the sweet spot inside my pussy is intense, and I know he must be enjoying the view of my ass as I ride him, must be feeling so frustrated that he can't touch my cheeks with his hands. I keep one hand on his thigh to steady myself as I rock back and forth, and the other to rub myself – the whole area between my legs is deliciously wet.

'I'm touching myself,' I tell him between my heavy breaths. 'Too bad you can't.'

His moans crescendo as I continue to move, and so do mine, and within seconds we've both crumpled into ecstasy.

I lay down beside him, my body pressed up against his, my pussy still pulsing, listening to the sounds of his breath become slower. And, like a good boy, he eventually falls asleep. That's my cue. I dress silently and step out of the cell, closing the door of it ever so quietly as I do so. The cherry on the cake is that, as I turn the lock for good measure, I see the gold watch sticking out of the sheriff's trouser pocket strewn on the floor. I reach carefully down and grab it. And with that, I disappear into the night.

Fingers crossed he catches me again.

TIP 16:

BUTT STUFF

An increasing number of vulva owners are having anal sex, but for lots of others there's a certain trepidation around it. If you're curious, solo anal play can be an amazing way to start exploring that area of pleasure. It's worth reminding yourself that millions of people do anal, and for a good reason! It's not dirty, it's actually very pleasurable.

Before delving into anal play you might need to prep a little more than you would for other internal penetration. The best time to trial anal is after the notorious 'ghost poo' – those times where you wipe and there is nothing there. However, let's not get too caught up in needing to be squeaky clean; if you're delving into the bum then there is going to be shit, and that's okay! Just like vaginal discharge, we have other bodily fluids that we have no need to be ashamed about. Just make sure that you personally feel prepped and comfortable so you're keen to explore, and that you wash your hands thoroughly afterwards.

Before inserting anything make sure you have used lots of lube (see page 66), the more the better for anything anal.

I'd suggest trying fingers or small butt plugs at first and then you can work your way up to bigger toys. Make sure you're using anal toys that have a base that won't go disappearing up inside you. Not to scare you, but this is really important as our anal muscles love to suck things up inside.

Sometimes penetration down here alone can be enough if you're touching yourself in other places too, but if you do want to explore more movement remember to start slowly and work your way up, always making sure you're being safe for your body. For example, you might start out with a rocking motion rather than pulling in and out, or simply pushing in a bit deeper. To build up you could slowly pull out and push back in – if this feels good you can experiment with rhythm and speed. And I know I've already said it in this tip but here's another reminder: the more lube the better!

NOTE: You can buy anal training kits that come with various sizes so you can work your way up to the bigger ones. As above, make sure you're always using anal toys that have a base that will not go past your entry muscles.

PLUGGED
AND PUBLIC

READING TIME
<7 MINUTES

THE SEXUAL PARTNER IS
MISCHIEVOUS

SEXY CHECKLIST
☐ MASTURBATION
☐ CLIT PLAY/FINGERING
☐ CUNNILINGUS
☐ BLOW JOB
☐ NIPPLE PLAY
■ VAGINAL PENETRATION
■ ANAL/BUTT PLAY
☐ SPANKING
■ SEX TOYS
☐ CHOKING
■ BDSM

My phone lights up in the corner of the room, buzzing on my bedside table. I'm just out of the shower, so with my hands still wet, I leave it there, the blue glow of the screen flashing. I know it's him. Adrenalin starts coursing through my veins as I draw out the anticipation of reading his message, a flutter pinching between my legs. I realise I'm in too deep when just hearing my phone buzz makes me feel like I'm the one vibrating. We've been dating only a few weeks, but every time with him has been incredible. He is truly wild.

I read the message, too curious to keep away any longer:

> Meet me outside the station in town. 4pm. Wear what I left you last time I was around. See you then x

Just as I finish reading the message there's another buzz.

> Do not under any circumstances not wear it

As my senses heighten from the excitement, I rack my brain trying to remember if he left lingerie last time he was over. I flush as I clock what it was. It wasn't clothing, it was a butt plug. He wants me to wear a butt plug out in public. Why does the thought secretly thrill me? I know it feels so good having it in during sex, but I can't imagine walking around in it. The hidden secret in my pants . . . sounds kind of hot.

There he is, waiting outside the station. I tense my butt cheeks without thinking, making me all the more aware of what I have been travelling in. As I walk over to him I can feel the fullness in my ass and yet the twinge of pleasure is in my pussy. All the people wandering around, going about their days completely oblivious to our little secret.

He winks at me as I approach, pulls me into an embrace and leans close to my neck. 'Did you do as I told you?'

His voice sends small shocks of pleasure down my body, radiating to the plug in my ass without him so much as touching me.

'It's in,' I say, trying to restrain my big smile before it becomes a giggle.

'Excellent,' he says. 'Let's go have dinner.'

Part of me wants to complain, to say – *Er, I've had a butt plug in my ass for half an hour now; I want you to fuck me already.* But I know the wait will intensify the pleasure, the not knowing when I'll get what I want is half the fun.

He takes my hand and leads me down the high street. With each step I take the plug is undeniably there, I am filled to capacity, it presses on the back wall of my pussy. I'm imagining what it's going to be like in a restaurant, how much the feeling will escalate when I'm sitting down, whether the waiting staff will notice as I move my weight from ass cheek to ass cheek, the sighs I'll exude every time I try to cross my legs. As the anticipation rises, he moves his hand to the small of my back and slides us down a narrow alleyway between a cosmetics shop and a restaurant. The bustling chatter of the tables from out front fades slightly as we walk further down the deserted path – there's a fire-exit door to the restaurant with a couple of bins next to it, but nothing else except the brick wall at the end.

'Where are we going?' I ask.

'Change of plan.' His lips curl into a mischievous grin. 'I want you right here, right now.'

My eyes dart around the alley. We've passed the restaurant's fire exit, we're near the brick wall at the bottom, but there's still only 20 metres between us and the people ambling past on the high street.

'Right here?' I bite my lip. My pussy throbs and makes my butt plug all the more obvious to me.

'Exactly,' he says. 'Underneath the noses of All. These. People.'

He pushes me against the wall, kissing me deeply on my mouth, his tongue boldly encircling mine. My breath catches in my throat, my heart racing as I realise that this is happening. I've already made up my mind but I say, because I feel I probably should, 'What if people see us?'

He shrugs. 'So what if they do?' He smiles conspiratorially at me before diving into my neck to bite me. I gasp as his teeth grip onto my skin, the little bubbles of pain shooting shockwaves through me. Each one sends pulses into my ass where the butt plug is, and it heightens the pleasure.

I pull him towards me, my adrenalin soaring, and as I get lost in our passionate kiss with my eyes closed, I forget where we are just enough to lose my inhibitions, but still make sure to keep my ear trained on the chatter of the people sat outside the restaurant and the footsteps of the people on the street. Knowing people are nearby is so very hot.

He puts his hand between my legs to feel me, and then reaches further back to feel *it*. I tense at his warm touch through the fabric of my knickers. He moves his fingers over the hard round edge of the plug, pushing at it, plunging it in even further. I whimper with pleasure as he moves my knickers aside and puts his fingers to my lips, teasing my entrance and then circling my clit. I bite on to his neck to stifle the sounds of my moans. He uses both hands to pull my knickers down, so far that they fall the rest of the way to my ankles. Then his rough hands tug up the skirt of my dress, completely exposing me. He unzips his jeans but doesn't pull them down; instead, he reaches inside the fly of his boxers so his hard cock can spring out.

I shoot a glance down the alley, seeing the people still walking by in the distance, the adrenalin from being so exposed making me feel almost high. I realise that not only do I enjoy the fact that they're there – I *want* somebody to see.

He grabs my chin and moves me to face him, his eyes sticking to mine. He spits on his hand and moves it over his cock and around the lips of my pussy. The tease makes my breath quicken. My heart beats hard in my chest waiting for him to push himself in. 'You're so hot, I want everybody to see that I get to fuck you,' he breathes in my ear as he bends his knees slightly and plunges his cock deep inside me. I take a sharp inhale as he fills me up. He's exactly the right height to make this work, our pelvises perfectly aligned, but it feels different to how it normally does because we're standing up, because of the plug – it's a tighter, fuller experience.

'Can you feel your plug?' he asks.

'Yes, yes I can!' I breathe heavily. The plug stretches my anus wide, intensifying the sensation of him fucking me as he pushes himself deeper into me.

'I knew you'd like it,' he says. He pulls at my hair so that I look at him. We fuck like that, staring deeply into each other's eyes as he pulls out and pushes in. I stand on my tiptoes so my pelvic floor tightens around him and moan loudly at the intensity of the pleasure, completely forgetting about our location, starting to register that I can't take much more. He pushes his hand over my mouth and then slows down abruptly, pushing me harder against the wall. His cock pushing in deeper. His face turned away from me.

I follow his gaze. A waiter has stopped dead in his tracks by the restaurant back door. He's gawping at us, seemingly unable to move. My heart is racing, and I'm even more turned on now that we've been caught, making my pussy tighten all the more on his cock. He tenses too, responding to me. I put my hands around the back of his neck and pull him into me, and he moves the pace up a notch as I continue looking at the stranger. I can feel my pulse throughout my whole body, my ass cheeks tighten around the plug, my climax builds, his breath is heavy and hard on my cheek, the waiter unable to tear his eyes away from us.

He cums inside me and as soon as he's done he reaches his hand down and rubs my wet clit. I only need him to touch it for ten seconds before I'm cumming too. I let out a primal moan – *'Fuck!'* – and as I close my eyes with the power of it, I see the waiter dart back inside.

He kneels down to where my pants are, helps shimmy them up my legs and back into place. He kisses me on the mouth. We both laugh a little, disbelieving of what we've just done. Then he nods at the restaurant door. 'Now let's go have dinner.'

ASK AROUND

One of my main missions in life is to normalise having conversations about sex. Not just the romance of it, but the actual nitty-gritty stuff that we usually feel too embarrassed to say out loud. What I've always found quite strange is that even when I started talking about sex with friends over maths textbooks at the back of class, we never spoke about masturbation. I remember us going so far as talking all about condoms, the different ones we'd tried (pleasure max, ribbed) and how the sensations varied. But we didn't ever think to talk about touching ourselves, even though we were probably all doing it once a day (it was puberty, after all).

For some reason (I mean, it's so clearly society, religion and all of that) we still feel too embarrassed and ashamed to talk about how we can make ourselves feel in our adult life. Personally, I was shrouded in the fear of what people might say or think if I brought it up for over half my life – until I met my best friend Reed. When Reed and I became friends we instantly connected over our excitement and enthusiasm for sex. She was the first person I'd ever had such open conversations with. We spoke about EVERYTHING. We normalised nipple hair, discharge, kinks *and* masturbation . . . all by just having a conversation together where one of us could reply: 'OMG, me too!'

The power of talking to your friends is immeasurable – not only does it eradicate shame and insecurities you have, you can learn so much as well. Your mate might have tried a new technique you never thought of before, or have a really hot fantasy that could make you wetter than ever! I know I'm making it sound really easy. Talking about masturbation could be quite a scary thing depending on your friendship group and cultural or religious background, and you don't want to make anybody you love feel uncomfortable. But I'm positive there is at *least* one person you know who wants you to bring it up to them, and honestly, once you've popped the cherry you will not be able to stop.

So for this tip, my suggestion is – call up or text your friend and ask them what they last did when they masturbated. Or you could start the conversation by bringing up sex toys – which ones have they tried? Do they have any specific recommendations? How do they use that?!

And give a little back. You know what would be a shame? Keeping all these amazing tips you're learning about your own body as you progress through this book to yourself. You can also help normalise conversations about masturbation by being honest when you've done it. If tomorrow your friend asks you what you got up to yesterday – tell them you had mind-blowing solo sex. 'I had an amazing shower and then I slipped into bed and made love to myself . . . '

To prove the benefits of all this talking, before I started writing this tip I texted Reed to ask her when the last time she masturbated was and how she did it. She's a speedy replier, so here's her response:

Well well well, I treated myself to a full wank sesh just two nights ago. I made sure this new sex toy was all charged up; it's been quite the pleasurable addition to my extensive collection. It's a dual-pleasure toy (clitoral and G-spot stimulation) – I lubed it up and decided to have a nice slow play. Although the good old trusty porn videos made the end come much quicker than anticipated, I had such a deep long orgasm which was extremely satisfying.

Obviously my next question was – what is this amazing sex toy?! But also her answer proves other things that some people might find comforting to hear: that it's okay to watch porn, that if you yourself cum super quickly while watching it then other people do too, and that the combo of sex toy plus porn might just produce top-notch orgasms.

Conversely, an answer like this might make you feel a bit prudish; like your own masturbation routine isn't hot enough. So to quash that, I also asked her if that's a typical masturbation moment for her. She answered:

> Normally when I masturbate, it's late at night, minutes before I turn my light off to sleep. There is usually no porn, just my imagination and the best sex toy ever created: the wand. I reach a clitoral orgasm in about 5–10 mins and then, covered in sweat, I place the wand back under the bed and go to sleep happy.

This is very similar to what I do about 80 per cent of the time, which has what effect? It makes me feel NORMAL. So go on – ask around. I'm sure you'll learn something new and it'll make you feel really comfortable about all this masturbating you're doing.

I have one last, slightly crazy, idea for you on this theme. How about taking THIS book to your next book club, and having a group conversation on masturbation? Wild, I know. But imagine the empowerment of a conversation like that!

MY FIRST SEX PARTY

READING TIME

>10 MINUTES

THE SEXUAL PARTNER IS

AN EXCITING STRANGER

SEXY CHECKLIST

- ■ MASTURBATION
- ■ CLIT PLAY/FINGERING
- ■ CUNNILINGUS
- ■ BLOW JOB
- ☐ NIPPLE PLAY
- ■ VAGINAL PENETRATION
- ☐ ANAL/BUTT PLAY
- ☐ SPANKING
- ☐ SEX TOYS
- ☐ CHOKING
- ■ BDSM

As I walk up to the venue my map app is pointing to, I look around the warehouse district wondering whether the people having food at the brewery next door are aware of what's happening right under their noses. If they stop chatting, would they hear the sound of a hundred people entangled together, of flesh being caressed or slapped in unison, of multiple orgasms raising the roof at the same time? In truth, I don't know if that *is* what's happening. I gulp, looking up at the large, windowless steel building. This is my first ever sex party.

I clutch my coat around me to hide the little clothing I have underneath. I'm wearing black fishnets and a thong, with a mesh top that exposes my nipples. You don't come to something like this wearing nice jeans and a top. If you're in, you're all in.

I join the queue to get inside; all the people within it seem to be buzzing with the same anticipation I'm feeling. My mind continues to race with the possibilities of what I'll find when I reach the door. I can't tell if the butterflies swarming in my stomach are making me feel nauseous . . . or playful.

The queue is sifted through the entry system; bags are checked, we're told where to find everything and the rules of the party are read out. Consent willingly given, we're allowed to stream inside. My eyes are immediately stimulated in every single direction. I'm in a sort of open-air courtyard, and around the outside bar is a mess of congregating bodies wearing little to nothing. Think festival attire but even less material. There is kink wear, bondage belts, latex and leather straps. Lace and lingerie and stockings. Bare breasts and ass cheeks jiggle as people walk, laugh and flirt.

I find my way on to the dance floor. My senses are flooded in all aspects – throbbing music blaring from speakers with a DJ in nothing but briefs, the smell of hot bodies, the dry ice hovering in the air highlighted by white spotlights beaming down, also lighting up people's writhing, dancing bodies. It's the sort of scene you usually see in slow-mo in a movie. I'm transfixed by everything – everyone seems so free. There is a horniness in the air and it's impossible not to catch it.

I start to dance, letting my hands explore my body in a way I'd never do in a normal club. A male voice announces himself from over my shoulder. My heart skips as I turn. He's hot, wearing the tiniest shorts I've ever seen.

He introduces himself and extends his hand. A formal handshake seems funny at a sex party. I smile and take it, introducing myself to him.

'Do you want me to show you where to put your coat?' he shouts over the music.

I look down; I'd forgotten I was still wearing it. I nod. He takes my hand – I notice how it feels in a way I wouldn't normally. Not too soft, not too rough, warm, firm and comforting. He takes me to the cloakroom – there's a long queue but over here I can hear him more easily. We swap stories of how we got here and laugh about what our neighbours would have thought if they'd seen our outfit choices. Then we start talking about *why* we're here. The atmosphere between us changes as we say what we like. What we think we might like if we tried it.

I hand over my coat to the cloakroom attendant. We move to some seats nearby and my new friend roams his eyes over my legs barely concealed by the fishnets, and the mesh top that shows off my breasts. He smiles appreciatively. 'You look . . . ' he says, and smiles harder. I feel a tingling sensation from being under his gaze. 'Can I kiss you?' he asks and leans closer. A rush of adrenalin sweeps through my veins.

I nod. He's already told me he likes direct eye contact, that it heightens sensations for him, so I keep my eyes on his. I told him I like the pain when someone pulls my hair; he goes for it now – it tips my head back so that my mouth is offered up to him. He leans in and presses his lips to mine and I move into him, slipping my tongue into his mouth. I'm suddenly in a trance with this man, the surrounding people and the beat of the music from the nearby dance floor blur out and it's just me and him. As he pulls away, the reality of where we are rushes back in and the sight of two people next to us passionately kissing, their tongues so obviously exploring each other's mouths, makes me want more. I can't help but giggle at the suddenness of this encounter, but I'm here to follow my desires. And I do.

I tell him I haven't been to the playroom yet; does he want to check it out? He says he'd love to. He takes my hand again and leads me towards a metal staircase. He lets me go up first so that he can have the view of my bum in the fishnets and thong I'm wearing. I exaggerate my movements as I walk up the stairs.

We're on a balcony that runs all the way around the dance floor. We walk hand in hand to the room opposite us. We'd been told where it was when we arrived, but it's clearly signposted by the red light flooding from the doorway on to the dark walkway. As we near it, the sound of slapping and pleasure spills out towards us, mixing in with the music from downstairs. I notice I'm not feeling nervous. I want whatever's coming next.

I peer through the plastic sheets that are blocking the doorway, then pull us through. My eyes are met with scenes I have only ever imagined in my wildest fantasies. The room is full of apparatus I don't even know the names of. Someone's using a bench designed for spanking – padded leg holders keep her legs wide apart and her ass up in the perfect position. A man holds his hand raised and then forcefully smacks her ass with a loud slap that echoes through the room. There are railings that you can get tied up to or lean on to fuck standing up. Mats on the floor are covered in various bodies, some naked, some still in their get-up. Threesomes, foursomes and moresomes are writhing all over the room, with orgasmic moans that sound like sweet pleasurable music. In the corner, a woman is giving a man a sort of strip search, patting down his arms before running her hands very slowly from his ankles up to his thighs, where her hand disappears into his ass. Another woman is fucking herself with a dildo while she watches two guys make out in front of her. Wrapping around the room like clingfilm is the smell of massage oil, lube, sweat and cum. It's overwhelming and incredible all at the same time.

I spy a tall railing with cuffs hanging from the top.

'I want you to pin me against that and kiss me,' I tell him. The corners of his lips turn up and he tells me that I'm a good girl for asking for that. The room is hot from all the fucking bodies, but the hard metal is cold against my exposed skin and juts into my body. His hands push on me and he stares deep into my eyes; they glow in the red light of the room. There is an intensity between us as we stand there staring into each other. He leans in and slips his tongue into my mouth.

'I want you to touch yourself,' he says, pulling back. I obey by sucking on my finger so it's wet and then slipping a hand into my knickers to rub my clit back and forth.

'Good girl,' he says, keeping his eyes fixed on mine. Heat floods my body as he watches me. He comes close to me and pulls my hair again. My pussy throbs as he controls me. He reaches into his shorts, pulls out his erect cock and starts stroking himself, all while gazing into my eyes. A moan releases itself from my throat, the heat between us building.

He leads us over to a wide, bed-like bench that already has two couples on either end mid-sex, moaning and thrusting. He tells me to sit down between them and I do, my eyes wandering over their bodies, fuelling my own horniness. He grips his cock in front of my face and pulls on my hair so I'm locking eyes with him again.

'Open your mouth,' he says. I do. He leans down slightly and lets a heavy drop of saliva fall from his mouth into mine. I take it on to my tongue, feeling a rush of blood in my cheeks.

'Good girl,' he says again. His orders and praise are turning me on way more than I was expecting. Maybe this is what I've needed all along. He releases my head and gestures to his cock. I take him into my mouth, opening wide to fit his girth between my lips, his warm shaft slipping over my tongue. I can feel that he likes it when I take his cock to the back of my throat. He groans as I pleasure him.

Then he pushes me back on to the bench, looking down at my pussy. My tights are in the way.

'Rip them,' he commands. I do as he says, tearing my fishnets open at the crotch ready for him. 'Good girl,' he says.

He pulls my knickers aside and spits into his hand to take his fingers inside me. I gasp at the feel of him, his warm hands cupping my lips as his fingers massage my G-spot. He leans down and sucks on my clit at the same time. I enjoy the feeling all the more by looking at the people to the left of me. A cock is travelling all the way out of a pussy slowly and then slamming back in again. As I watch, my hunger increases.

I look back down at him between my legs and put my hand on the top of his head. 'Fuck me,' I demand.

He wipes his mouth with a hand and moves over me, his body looking spectacular in the red light. He kisses me and I taste myself on his tongue. There are condom boxes all over the room; he goes to grab one, returning through the maze of naked, grinding bodies, and slides it on to his hard cock while I lay back on the bench. I touch myself in anticipation, circling my fingers around my clit. I hold my knickers to the side as he leans over me and slides his rock-hard cock into me. I gasp as he slowly, inch by inch, pushes in deeper. My pussy throbs around his thick shaft. I'm instantly flooded with bolts of electricity from each thrust as he fills me up perfectly. I stare down at him pushing in and out and then back up into his eyes. He grabs my hair and holds my gaze.

'Touch yourself,' he says.

I reach down and circle my clit, which immediately tightens me around his cock.

'Good girl,' he says with a groan.

He looks to my right and I copy; a beautiful woman is being fucked from behind, her face in a euphoric expression as it's pressed into the bench. Her moans are entangling with my own.

I look back into his eyes as my pleasure builds and builds. His cock is hitting that special place and I can feel myself edging into climax as I continue to touch myself. He thrusts deeper and deeper and I can feel him throbbing inside me. **His hand grips tighter on my hair and a wave of heat washes over me. I let out a loud moan, loud enough to distract some of the other lovers in the room, as I orgasm in complete ecstasy. Adding to the room filled with pleasure.**

'Cum for me,' I beg.

His eyes twinkle at my order and he obeys. Groaning deeply as I feel him pulsing inside me, releasing himself completely.

He collapses on to me and I smile widely into his shoulder.

I just got fucked at a sex party, among all these other people. Life truly is wild.

Now to see what the rest of the night might entail . . .

TIP 18:

EDGING

Do you know what feels better than an orgasm? An orgasm that you denied yourself a few times over. Why not use the next story to give it a go?

Edging, or orgasm control, might already be a common practice for you during partnered sex. But it can also be used for incredible results within solo sex and masturbation. Edging is when you build yourself up to orgasm, but just before you lean over that edge, you take away stimulation and stop the orgasm from happening. It's a really amazing way to build pleasure and extend your experience. You can deny yourself orgasm as many times as you want and then when you're ready to push over the edge the pleasure is usually way higher than it would have been in the first case.

My suggestion when you're trying this out is to press your hands down firmly on to your vulva in a cupping position just before you think you're about to orgasm – don't just remove your hands completely as taking away the sensation can be too thrilling a sensation in itself! The number of times you deny yourself is up to you but if you're just starting out, perhaps try denying yourself twice and then cumming on the third time so you can make sure you don't frustrate yourself.

FYI some vibrators have settings that are similar to edging, where they build up to a higher vibration and speed and then start back at the beginning again.

NOTE: It can take some practice to master the timing for orgasm control and edging, so don't beat yourself up if you lose your orgasm completely or have a petite one instead – make sure you're enjoying the experience and not putting pressure on yourself to cum.

I SPY

READING TIME
>10 MINUTES

THE SEXUAL PARTNER IS
COMBATIVE

SEXY CHECKLIST
☐ MASTURBATION
☐ CLIT PLAY/FINGERING
■ CUNNILINGUS
■ BLOW JOB
☐ NIPPLE PLAY
■ VAGINAL PENETRATION
☐ ANAL/BUTT PLAY
☐ SPANKING
☐ SEX TOYS
■ CHOKING
☐ BDSM

I remove my eye from the free-standing telescope because my leg is going numb and I need to shake it awake. Lying on any concrete roof is uncomfortable, but lying on a Moscow concrete roof in March is *freezing*. I'm wearing thermals under my all-in-grey get-up (to camouflage as best I can into this abandoned office block) – but it doesn't matter how much you've got on: if you're not moving, you're going to get cold. *I wish he'd go back to Panama*, I think to myself – trailing him there was lovely.

I put one eye back to the telescope. It's trained seven storeys below, at the smart café across the road which he always frequents when he's here. (Rookie error that – having a routine.) I can see that he's stirring his coffee with one hand, leafing through a paper with the other. 'He' is a hot-shot Russian lawyer, working for an oligarch who's been trading in illegal firearms. He turned double agent for us years ago, but now we have reason to believe he's withholding important intelligence; that he may actually be using his position as mole to spy on us. My mission is to get proof one way or the other.

A waiter comes over to see if he wants any food. I know already that he'll send them away – he doesn't eat before noon. Watching someone so closely means you learn things about them. I know, for instance, that he likes jazz music, that he irons his own shirts rather than sending them out, that he finds it easy to pick up men or women from bars but that he never takes them home, only to hotel rooms, where he likes to fuck them against the windows. Just last night he was in the Four Seasons overlooking Red Square, passionately fucking a blonde woman while looking out over the Kremlin. I think he must like good views.

He drains his coffee and throws some change onto the table, putting his gloves and coat on. As he walks out of the café and away down the road, I marvel that he doesn't need to button up his coat, but I keep my eye trained on the table. He's left the newspaper there; it's not a very 'him' move and I wonder if he could have stowed something inside it for somebody to come and collect. I wait to see if anybody arrives but nobody does. I bite my lip, thinking. The café is only across the street and the waiting staff are slow. I might have time to get over there and make sure for myself.

Quick as a flash I take apart the telescope, pack it into my rucksack and head to the stairwell. The rusty metal door clanks as I open it. I start to descend . . . when a chill washes over my body. There's a sort of prickle at the back of my neck that makes me think someone else might be nearby. I stop, my senses going into overdrive, straining my ears to see if I can hear anything. But I see and hear nothing and I need to get to the café, so I set off again.

Moving was a mistake. Before I'm able to take a second step, I've been slammed into the wall by someone appearing from the shadows behind me. A forearm juts into my throat, almost cutting off my oxygen and making me unable to move. I can't believe it. It's *him*.

'Why are you following me?' he shouts in English with a thick Russian accent.

FUCK. I swallow, mind whirring fast as I try to create a cover story.

He grabs my jaw with his leather-gloved hand. It's weird seeing him this close in real life – normally I'm zooming in on him from afar. His eyes are cold, but they're fascinatingly piercing. His fingers pinch into my cheeks as he says again, *'Why are you following me?'*

'I'm not,' I say, attempting to sound scared – which isn't hard to fake as it's true. 'I don't know who you are – I'm just a contractor for a property developer, I'm doing a survey.' I cough dramatically from the pressure of his arm on my throat, hoping it'll make me seem innocently pathetic.

He laughs, a proper cackle. I suddenly clock that he's talking to me in English and my stomach drops. How did he know I wasn't Russian? 'That's very good,' he says, 'but I know exactly who you are, *Special Agent Clark.*'

Time to go. I launch my knee into his balls. He crumples and I jump down the steps four at a time, swinging around the rails. My heart is beating out of my chest, racing in fear and excitement. If I'm honest, this adrenalin is why I love my job so much.

Loud claps on the stairs behind me tell me he's up and in hot pursuit. I'm small and nimble, he's taller and bulkier – I know I have the advantage – but I chance a glance back to see where he is. It means I don't see the broken stair in front of me and I crash into the floor, pain blooming from the spot I land on.

Two hands haul me down to the next landing and then he uses his knees to pin down my thighs, restraining my hands by pushing them down together on my chest. I battle against him in vain as he asks me again: 'Why are you following me? Tell me and I'll think about letting you go.'

Clearly he's had training on how to fight, but I know he's a businessman at heart and no businessman likes spit in his eye. I pool my saliva and launch it at him. He pulls his hands off me immediately so he can wipe his face, freeing my elbow to launch it into his ribs. He doubles over in pain but, try as I might to push him off my legs, he won't move them and I'm still stuck. I try another tactic. I reach my hands into his coat, feeling his warm, solid chest beneath my hands as I find my way to his armpits – and I tickle him. This time it works. He recoils and I can push him off me. I launch myself down the next flight of stairs, adrenalin working my legs so hard I feel almost like I'm flying.

Then I feel a hand on the back of my rucksack pulling me back. I try to slip my arms from out of the loops but too late. He's got me again. He slams me against the wall once more, this time pushing his knees up against my thighs so I can't move my leg to hurt his balls. His face is an inch from mine, his breath hot on my face, and his cock – his rock-hard cock – is pressing into me.

I cast my eyes downwards to check I'm right. I am. 'This doing it for you?' I say malevolently. The truth is . . . it's kind of doing it for me. I love the adrenalin of being chased so much that I can feel I'm wet inside my pants. I continue, hoping to embarrass him – men with big egos hate that: 'I thought you only liked doing it when you have a good view.'

He laughs coldly again. 'You think you're so clever,' he says, his eyes dropping to my lips, his expression one of abject anger mixed with a deepening desire. He leans forward and whispers into my ear. 'I do it by the window so that you'll see me.'

All along he's known I've been watching him. Fear and pleasure tingle down my spine in equal measure. I struggle against him, but now I realise I'm not trying to escape – it's because by fighting him, I can feel his cock rubbing into my crotch all the more.

I can't help it: following my own desires I lean forward and kiss him hard on the lips. He kisses me back, moving his tongue into my mouth so boldly that saliva is pushed out of it. He pulls back and licks it up, pausing to look into my eyes again. 'Undo my belt,' he commands.

He releases his weight on me just enough so that my arms, pinned to my sides, can undo the buckle. I undo the button and zip too and push his trousers down so that they fall the rest of the way. He pulls back from me but pushes my shoulders down. 'Get on your knees and suck it,' he says. Slowly, so he doesn't have any reason to fear what I'm doing, I do as he says. Once on my knees, I wriggle down his briefs and his cock springs out. I can't believe I'm doing this. Anticipation surging through me, I deepthroat it into my wet mouth. It feels incredible – long and hard and as if it would fill my pussy completely.

He keeps his hands on my shoulders but as he relaxes into it, my chance comes. With my free hands I slip the belt out of his fallen trousers, double it over and whip it up between his legs with a satisfying 'thwack' so that it bites into his bare ass.

He cries out in pain and it gives me the chance to push him down the remaining step to the next landing, where he falls on his back. While he's stunned, I use the opportunity to drop my grey trousers and thermals and to sit my wet pussy directly down onto his hard cock. I gasp with the pleasure of it as it fills me up, and I rock up and down on him, shooting sparks of pleasure making me tighten around him. The friction of his cock inside my pussy makes me want to melt, to sit here, bouncing up and down on him for ever. Then I see his hand reaching into his coat pocket – for a gun, for a knife? I can't risk finding out. I grab his throat, continuing to ride him as I constrict his airways, so his hands have to give up with what they were searching for and try to peel off my wrists instead.

He can't manage that, but with an incredible surge of strength he pushes me up and off his cock, flipping me over so I'm on my back. He plummets his cock back into me and I scream out in ecstasy. He pulls out and pushes in so that I feel drastically empty and then completely full up. Now he moves *his* hands to *my* throat. The dizzying lack of air makes the pleasure of him filling me up all the more intense – I don't even try to push him off.

'Giving up already,' he says mockingly between heavy pants, goading me as he pounds me.

The good thing about him choking me is that he can't control my arms. I wrap them around his back and dig my fingernails in. He shouts out in pain and his hands release from my throat as he sits up away from me. I rock myself up to sitting too and push him back down on his back again. Moving quickly, I crawl up his body so that I can straddle his neck with my thighs, knees on the cold concrete floor, and plant my wanting pussy down on his mouth. I rest my thumbs under his eyes and tell him that I'll hurt him if he makes a wrong move. He doesn't say anything because he can't. Instead, he looks up at me with those cold eyes as he laps his warm tongue over my clit. I'm determined to cum this way, for me to take my pleasure without him getting his. My climax builds as he rolls his tongue all over me. He licks my lips, pushes inside my pussy and then circles around and over my clit again. Around and over, around and over until it sends me into spirals. **I close my eyes, I lean into him, and pleasure erupts through me.**

As soon as I orgasm he knows I'm at my weakest. He ducks out from underneath me, rolls himself over and pushes me face down into the concrete landing. With his hand pressed on my back he slips his cock into me and fucks me harder and harder from behind. With a huge shudder and a moan, he cums.

He collapses his weight on top of me and for a few moments we both lie there, still and silent. Then I try to move, but he keeps me pinned down.

'I still need to know why you're following me,' he breathes heavily into my ear.

Looks like we're going to do this all over again.

FLIRT WITH ALL FIVE OF YOUR SENSES

We touched a little on sensory play earlier with temperature and texture, but for this tip I want to encourage you to really think about how you're going to activate all five of your senses as you read the next story.

TOUCH

What are you using to touch yourself? Hands, vibrators, glass or other toys?

SOUND

What are you hearing? Maybe you're listening to this book! But if you're reading it, then is there a sexy soundtrack on the speakers or do you want to look on YouTube for relaxing noises, like rain on a window, rainforest sounds or birdsong?

SIGHT

Where are you and what can you see? If you're listening to this book, do you want to look at sexy imagery at the same time? Maybe today it would turn you on most to sit by a window and look out over your garden if you have one? Or maybe it's about the mood lighting.

SMELL

Do you have any incense or a candle you can light that will turn you on? Do you have a favourite perfume that makes you feel irresistible? Do you have a yummy-smelling body lotion you can lather yourself with?

TASTE

If you were having sex with somebody other than yourself, there's a chance you might have eaten or drunk something nice with them. Indulge yourself during solo sex too! What would you like to taste on your tongue while you touch yourself? Would chocolate get you in the mood? A sip of wine? Strawberries? Or pizza?!

It's really worth maximising all of your senses during solo sex; if we give focus to all of them then we'll feel really awake to all of the sensations coming our way, and that awareness can heighten our pleasure.

AN OUTSIDE ORGASM FOR THREE

READING TIME

<10 MINUTES

THE SEXUAL PARTNERS ARE

NAUGHTY

SEXY CHECKLIST

■ MASTURBATION

■ CLIT PLAY/FINGERING

■ CUNNILINGUS

□ BLOW JOB

■ NIPPLE PLAY

■ VAGINAL PENETRATION

□ ANAL/BUTT PLAY

□ SPANKING

□ SEX TOYS

□ CHOKING

□ BDSM

I am woken up by the sun lapping at my bedcovers. I'm a proper sun baby, but living in a city isn't the best for soaking up the rays. Still, the blue sky looks so inviting . . . maybe I'll find a nearby park, put my new bikini on and get some vitamin D.

Before I go I stand naked in front of my mirror and apply suncream, pouring it out into my hand and rubbing it firmly and slowly all over my body. I catch myself in the reflection and pause in appreciation. I'm really feeling myself today. As I leave the house, pulling my shades on, the sun hits my face as if I'm dipping into a bath. The feeling of warmth and the self-confidence that I've woken up with today makes me feel content, relaxed – and maybe also ready for adventure.

The park isn't as busy as I thought it would be on a day like today; there are only a few groups of friends laying about on the grass listening to music, reading books, chatting away. I wander about looking for the perfect spot, somewhere secluded so I feel totally comfortable with showing a bit more flesh than your average day. I see a little clearing past a couple of big trees and bushes. Perfect! My own secret garden.

I strip down to my bikini: it's white with a cherry pattern on it, a little retro moment. After spreading my blanket on the ground I stretch out in the sunshine and let out a deeply contented sigh. This is my happy place. With the trees around me, the other people in the park are muted; I can only hear the rustle of the leaves as they brush against each other.

I close my eyes and fall into a daydream about a colleague . . .

when a giggle and a low voice startle me out of my daydreaming daze. Unsure of how I feel about people intruding on my secluded area, I sit up and turn over. Luckily my shades hide my curious eyes. It's an attractive couple. The woman is undressing, dropping a floaty peach dress to the ground as her boyfriend lays a picnic blanket down. To my surprise, she's stripping down to her underwear, which is in fact, just a very tiny thong revealing a round juicy bottom – and no bra to speak of. Her boyfriend is eyeing her with a grin on his face . . . and then he looks over to me. I quickly turn my head to face the other way and pretend I wasn't looking at them. My heart is racing; I've accidentally become a voyeur to their sexy, sunny afternoon. I want to look back but I don't . . . yet. Instead, I listen to them laughing and flirting. I can hear playful slaps and pretend bites and squeals. Then it goes quiet.

I turn my head as inconspicuously as I can to face them. The boyfriend, who is sitting down by the girlfriend's feet, is slowly tracing his hand over her body. Then he gets on all fours and starts kissing her from her toes all the way up her legs and stops, hovering over her thong. I can almost imagine his breath, warm, wanting on her skin. I'm sure they're going to catch me gawping at them but I can't look away. Anticipation is sweeping over me – are they going to continue this right here, right now, in front of me?

He pulls at her thong playfully with his teeth until she grabs his neck and encourages him to move up to her breasts. He starts by cupping them with his hands and then kisses them passionately. I can see his tongue circling her nipples and she arches her back as he sucks on them. My mouth opens and a little breath of pleasure echoes across the clearing. They both turn their heads and look at me. My first thought isn't embarrassment – it's disappointment. Now they've been caught, they'll stop and I don't want them to.

But then, surprisingly, they turn back to each other and start to kiss hungrily. Does this mean they want me to watch? No. I've got my sunglasses on – maybe, because I didn't say anything, they thought I wasn't looking at them and that's why they're carrying on. I force myself to stop watching – it feels too rude; I don't even know them! I lay my head back down on my blanket and close my eyes. Let them do what they want to do. I don't need to listen to them, to the wet sounds of their lips on each other's skin or the moans they elicit. The sun is so nice. I feel so warm. I feel so fucking horny.

The moans stop. I don't dare look at what they're doing now. But then—

I sense a shadow has fallen over my face. I prop myself up on my elbow and lift my shades. The girlfriend crouches down beside me completely naked, her breasts, directly in my eyeline, swinging to stillness. She is beautiful, her lips moist and eyes sparkling in the sunlight. The confidence of walking over to a stranger completely naked makes her so much more captivating.

'I saw you watching us,' she says.

I stare at her, my mouth open, unable to make words come out.

'We liked it . . . ' she continues.

'You did?' I breathe.

'Yes! We think you're really sexy. And . . . thought we'd ask if you'd like to come and join us?' She pauses, biting her lip. 'Don't worry if not; it's just you're really cute and it could be fun . . . '

I swallow. 'Wow. Um. I've really never done anything like that before,' I stutter.

'That's okay. ' She smiles naughtily at me. 'I'm going to go back to my boyfriend but if you feel like joining us, just come over.'

She stands up and goes back to their blanket. Her bum kind of bounces as she walks. He grabs it and pulls her down to him and she giggles. They are really fucking hot. Would it be totally mad to take them up on their offer? My heart is racing and I can feel my pussy throbbing, wanting, waiting for me to make a decision.

I look down at my own blanket and then back to them. They're making out now. He has his hand down the front of her thong and she's kissing his neck. Okay. I'm going to do it. As I stand up, a dog barks in the distance and I'm reminded we're in a park, not a bedroom. The thrill of a dog walker stumbling across us, as we might be tangled together, ignites more of a fire inside me. Every step I take towards them I feel my inhibitions disappearing. If they can do this, then, fuck it, so can I.

I reach their blanket, holding my breath slightly as I drop to my knees. They turn to me grinning, welcoming me. There's no soft initiation – the first thing they do is pull me into a gentle three-way kiss. Our tongues intermingle together, deliciously wet. We draw closer together – she's wearing a floral perfume, there's a hint of sweet sweat on him. Now that we're closer, tentatively I reach out a hand and place it on her body. Her skin is warm and soft. I follow the curve of her waist, wanting to touch her breasts but not feeling able to just yet.

We stop kissing each other because she's pulled away. I realise it's so she can concentrate on undoing my bikini top; it slides off me on to the blanket. Both their stares caress my breasts and my nipples, hungrily looking down to my bikini bottoms that have yet to come off. The boyfriend pushes me gently to lie on my back, moving his lips to my neck; his breath tickles and sends a shiver down my spine as his stubble brushes against my skin. His tongue lingers at my ear before softly kissing down to my nipples. He starts sucking and biting gently. Goosebumps bristle on my skin in pleasure. At the same time, the girlfriend kisses me on the mouth, sliding her tongue over mine deeply – almost invasively – so that I start to feel hungry for another hole of mine to be filled. As if she can read my mind she moves around her boyfriend, kissing him on his back as she works her fingers around my bikini bottoms. She pulls them down slowly, revealing my glistening pussy to the sky. I've never been naked outside before; feeling the sun on it feels incredible. The boyfriend stops tugging at my nipples with his teeth so he can take off his boxers, and I watch the girlfriend stand up and drop her thong to the floor. She picks it up, kneels beside my head and pops it in my mouth, as if to gag me. 'You might need this,' she said. It's such a hot thing to do, and I can taste her wetness on my tongue.

But now I'm in this, I want this. I throw the thong away, reach over and grab her arm, pulling her towards me. A grin curls at the corners of her mouth and she moves next to me, pressing her soft lips against mine, tickling my tongue with hers. Her boyfriend sits up between us and presses his fingers against both of our pussies. I feel my heart beating from between my legs. He teases the lips of my increasingly swollen vulva and encircles my clitoris with slow, light strokes, moving between the two in a teasing way. I moan into her mouth as the pleasure builds and the teasing gets more frustrating. She moves from my lips, down my neck, kissing, biting softly, breathing heavily on my skin. He stops touching me, making way for her to move between my legs, instead moving up to my head and kissing me deeply on the mouth. Just as I'm leaning into the sensation of his tongue in my mouth, I feel *her* tongue on my clit. Both the sensations happening at once are hypnotic. She takes my hand, pauses from sucking on my clit and guides my fingers into my pussy. It's so wet. She rubs my hand all over myself, then guides it towards her boyfriend's cock. It's warm and hard and I rub my wet hand over it. He moans quietly as I tighten my grip around him and gently move up and down.

'Do you want to fuck him?' the girlfriend asks.

I look over to him and he raises an eyebrow, hopefully, sexily, expectantly.

'Yes,' I breathe. 'I *really* want to fuck him.'

Expertly she tears open a condom packet she's pulled out of her bag. Watching her pull it on to his hard, alert cock is mesmerising, the supple slick sound it makes as it rolls down making me salivate. He lies down and she pulls me on top of him. His cock easily slips inside me. I lean backwards a little and want to shout out how good it feels, the warmth from the sun on my skin and the taste of fresh air in my mouth intensifying my enjoyment. The girlfriend crawls to his head and crouches her pussy over his mouth. She's opposite me, biting her lip. We're both rocking on him, letting him pleasure us. I grab her neck and pull her into a kiss. Moaning into each other's mouths in joint, mounting satisfaction. I've never felt so in tune with someone else's pleasure, it's like we're both building the orgasm together.

Waves of enjoyment are radiating from my pussy up into my mind. I can feel my muscles tightening, my breath getting shorter and faster. I feel so confident right now. I move my fingers to my clit. I can feel my orgasm building and building – I look at her opposite me and see from the expression on her face that it's the same for her. **His cock is hitting the perfect spot as I ride him, rocking back and forth. I can feel him reaching his climax, throbbing inside me. I let out a huge moan as my body is flooded with my own orgasm. It's the most intense pleasure I might have ever experienced. A joint ecstasy, a triple orgasm.** It's like the light from the sun is radiating through all of our bodies. We sparkle. And then we collapse to the blanket.

Not long afterwards, as I leave the park, my pussy still pulsing with what's just happened, I wipe a trickle of sweat off my neck with my finger. I suck on it. Tantalisingly, it could be mine, it could be his, it could be hers.

TIP 20:

STRIP BACK ALL SENSES

If you're reading chronologically it might seem odd that I'm talking about this given my previous tip was all about how to make sure you engage all five of your senses during solo sex. But bear with me! This tip is all about why it's worth taking some or all of them away.

If all you can sense is your touch, then the focus that provides could really heighten your pleasure. So try solo sex in silence in the dark. Using blindfolds (silk is nicest!) and noise-cancelling headphones can restrict senses in a way that feels pretty hot. Either way, when you can't hear or see anything, every other sense becomes heightened. Each touch is magnified. Experimenting with this can really help you get familiar with the texture of your body and the touches that you respond to.

For the next story, if you're reading this book then why not put earplugs in and only have the lights on low (or, if you have a partner, ask them to read it to you with a blindfold on too). If you're listening to this book then go for the eye mask.

Confession: I once masturbated in a float tank (100 per cent not allowed). If you don't know what that is, it's basically a little bath pod that encloses you in darkness and silence. You float in the salted water that keeps you on the surface, so when you lay back and relax it's like you're floating in space. The time I tried one of these out, I couldn't not experience such amazing sensory play! Needless to say, it felt amazing as I floated and touched myself.

BLINDFOLD ME

READING TIME

<10 MINUTES

THE SEXUAL PARTNER IS

SURPRISING

SEXY CHECKLIST

☐ MASTURBATION

■ CLIT PLAY/FINGERING

■ CUNNILINGUS

☐ BLOW JOB

■ NIPPLE PLAY

■ VAGINAL PENETRATION

☐ ANAL/BUTT PLAY

☐ SPANKING

■ SEX TOYS

☐ CHOKING

■ BDSM

He takes another mouthful of his steak, chewing it slowly while he waits for me to continue the conversation. I eye his lips, looking for something that will put me off even more, but he's actually chewing in quite a polite and inconspicuous manner.

'So, er, yeah, I guess at the moment I'm just looking to meet new people, make connections – maybe something will stick eventually but I'm not putting pressure on it . . . ' It's the usual waffle I repeat on dates in reply to the 'What are you looking for at the moment?' question. He finishes his mouthful and somehow looks arrogant without even saying anything. It's not his fault, really. I know I don't fancy these City types and yet I always say yes to going on dates with them.

My mind wanders on to thinking about the new Netflix thriller series I'm excited to watch when I get home, when he says, 'And what are you looking for . . . sexually?'

I raise my eyebrows. Not because I don't like articulating what I want, but because I'm not used to these kinds of men taking much interest in what I want in the bedroom. I look at him thoughtfully, liking where the conversation is going, but I'm considering how much information to give away to this stranger I've just met.

I opt for deflection: 'Why, what are *you* looking for?'

He grins at me. 'I have quite a specific desire. Are you interested in exploring your pleasure?'

What a question. 'I'm always interested in feeling *more* pleasure, if that's what you mean,' I say. He's intriguing me, though; maybe he's about to redeem our boring date?

'I really enjoy blindfolding women and getting to know their bodies in various different ways.' He pauses and looks at me intently to gauge my reaction at this news. I try to keep my face straight, but my mouth has fallen open slightly. 'If you'd be up for it, I'd like to take you home and blindfold . . . *you*.'

He lingers on the word 'you'.

I put my knife and fork together on the plate and say, as casually as I can, 'What would you do to me?'

'That would ruin the whole experience,' he says. 'If it's okay, I'd like you to trust me, and if there's anything you don't like you can say "red" and I'll stop right away.'

What the hell? I think. The Netflix series will have to wait.

He lives in a tall block of swanky modern flats. The typical bachelor pad – I wasn't expecting anything less – but it feels lived in: unfolded newspaper on the table, mugs waiting to go into the dishwasher, photographs of what must be family on the wall. It endears me to him. He puts his hands on my shoulders, which sends a rush of adrenalin through me, and then he leads me over to a door in the corner of the living room: his bedroom.

'This is where I'm going to blindfold you,' he says, closing the curtains at the window behind a large, grey-sheeted bed. 'Ready?'

'Ready,' I say. He's good at checking consent, which is hot, but the business-like way we've agreed this means I have to stop myself from laughing.

He goes to his bedside table and opens a drawer that is full of different objects I can't quite make out from where I'm standing by the door. He pulls out a black silk blindfold, the material sifting through his fingers seductively. I stop feeling the urge to laugh now; anticipation is prickling all the nerves in my body.

He goes behind me and drapes the blindfold over my eyes. I can't see anything. The material feels soft against the top of my cheeks and he ties it behind my head with the perfect tightness.

Taking my hand, he leads me to the bed. The touch of his skin on my fingers already feels more intense than it would if I could see. My heart is beating hard and fast, clueless to what is about to happen. The floor falls away from beneath me, and I realise it's because he's scooped me into his arms. He leans in close, his breath tickling my earlobe.

'I'm going to lay you down on the bed and undress you completely.' His voice softly plays at my ear, the vibrations from the sound causing goosebumps to prickle on my skin.

He does as he says, gently lying me down and then tenderly working the buttons on my dress out of their buttonholes. The movement of the fabric as it sifts over my skin shoots sparks over my chest and stomach. Each of his movements is slow, deliberate, and my breath is slow and steady to match it, feeling the full force of every sensation, including the anticipation and adrenalin that's fiercely begun to flow through me.

The cool air flushes over the top of my body as he suddenly whips the dress off from underneath me; the soft sheet I'm now lying on seduces my skin. He slips a hand under my back, unclips my bra and a moment later I hear it fall with a soft pat on the floor. I wonder what I look like to him – completely naked now except for my knickers. I know that must be where he's going next . . .

I feel his breath through the cotton material and my heart beats faster knowing that his head is between my legs. He teasingly traces over where my clit is with what must be his thumb, and then the pressure moves down to my pussy. I can feel his hot breath there too and I wish he'd pull my knickers aside and run his tongue over it. Instead, he bites and sucks at the inside of my thigh, his hands roaming up my legs. He stops and the absence of his touch when he pulls away sends shivers through me, not knowing what's going to come next. The unknown scares and excites me. I feel him hook his fingers into my knickers and he pulls them down and off. I'm now completely naked on the bed, at my most vulnerable, at his complete disposal.

I feel his weight shift on the bed and know he's got off it. I hear the drawer open next to me. The sound of clinking metal or maybe glass as he moves a couple of objects before retrieving what he wants. The slightest sound echoes around my head as I wait in anticipation.

A light tickling sensation erupts on my arm closest to him; he's draping something over me that feels almost as light as air but sends ripples over my entire body. It tickles a lot more than I was expecting, I bite my lip to stop myself from giggling. He moves the object up my arm and over my chest, down between my breasts, stopping to circle each one. My body squirms and bucks with the sensation that feels like a mixture of torture and pleasure at the same time. He moves it down to my feet. Oh *hell*. I gasp for air, trying to compose myself. I figure it must be a feather, which he then continues to move up my legs and slowly, so very slowly, towards my pussy. He brushes it past my lips and the sensation vanishes, only to be replaced with his wet tongue. The switch of sensations feels amazing, the light tease to the hard, warm, lapping tongue.

I dig my head back into the pillow and immerse myself in the hot, wet feeling of it. Then I notice there is a new object in play. It feels cold and hard as he moves it up the inside of my thigh. The chill of it makes me take a deep breath in. It feels weirdly perplexing, so smooth and almost silky gliding over my skin. He stops it at the entrance of my pussy, where it takes up the space between what I know must be my swollen and ready lips . . . but he doesn't move it any further. There's a longing inside me, wanting it to be pushed inside, impatient to understand its size and shape.

I gasp in surprise as now I hear a buzzing right next to my left ear. He moves the vibrator over my mouth, rests it on my lips, waiting for me to wet it with my tongue. 'Suck it,' he says – hearing his voice without seeing where he is makes my heart beat faster. I obey and take the vibrating object into my mouth and let my saliva cover it. My tongue tingles and I feel as if an electric current is running all the way through me.

'Good girl,' he says, the praise unexpectedly making me feel even more turned on. My pussy throbs: when will the mysterious object still resting on it be allowed to enter?

He moves the wet vibrator to my nipples and the buzzing tingles make them harden. Then he circles it around each breast rhythmically, my breathing getting heavier and deeper, and I know I could be on the edge fairly soon.

He traces the buzzing down to my clit, and just as a whimper leaves my mouth he pushes the cold, hard object he's kept at the entrance to my pussy deep inside me. I let out a loud moan that echoes around the room.

'Good girl,' he says again; I feel already as if I live to hear him say that. The object – which I can only presume is a glass or metal dildo – feels firm and wet inside me as he plunges it in and out, hitting my G-spot, while the vibrator sends thrills through my clit. Moaning, I twist my body around in the sheets, grabbing the material and squeezing it into fists; he is taking me to another level, pleasure like I've never experienced.

I can feel myself building up and up, the pleasure getting almost unbearable. My breath staggering.

Unsure of whereabouts he is, his next words seem to reverberate god-like around my head: 'You're going to cum for me now.'

He quickens the plunging dildo and moves the vibrator around in circular motions on my clit. Moans escape me without any ability to control myself.

'I'm going to cum,' I say.

'Good girl.'

And with that I'm sent into a whirlpool of warm orgasmic bliss. My pussy pulls the dildo deep inside me as I pulse around it. My body releases every inch of connection with the world for an amazing few seconds.

'You did really well. Thank you,' he says, his praises making me blush.

I never want to take the blindfold off.

MULTIPLE STIMULATION

When it comes to pleasure, sometimes one stimulation is enough, but often it can be a case of the more the merrier. Here are some variations to try out:

- Internal – clitoral

- Internal – clitoral –nipples

- Internal – clitoral – anal

- Clitoral – anal

- Internal – anal

- Clitoral – nipples

This is a good opportunity to find out what sensations heighten when you add more. Without clitoral stimulation you might not find as much pleasure internally, but when you add them both together it creates magic. This can be the same with all of your erogenous zones. Whether that's touching your inner thighs, nipples or using a butt plug! Things change and feel different when there is something else going on at the same time. Dual or even triple pleasure can be such an intense and amazing experience. For the next masturbation mediation, why not try out internal and clitoral, or clitoral and nipple play, at the same time. OR if you're feeling brave, internal, clitoral and anal! This definitely could be too much for some people, but if you're feeling adventurous it's a worthy expedition.

BETWEEN TWO COCKS

READING TIME
<7 MINUTES

THE SEXUAL PARTNERS ARE
CHEEKY

SEXY CHECKLIST
☐ MASTURBATION
■ CLIT PLAY/FINGERING
■ CUNNILINGUS
■ BLOW JOB
■ NIPPLE PLAY
■ VAGINAL PENETRATION
■ ANAL/BUTT PLAY
☐ SPANKING
☐ SEX TOYS
☐ CHOKING
☐ BDSM

On the sofa are my flatmate Daniel, our friend Reggie and me. I'm in the middle and we're snuggled up together because the boys have chosen an old classic horror to watch, of course. When I was a kid I absolutely terrified myself by watching *The Ring* – to this day I'm too freaked out to have a TV in my room. I don't know why the boys subject me to it. Sometimes I think it's just an excuse for them to cuddle up close to me.

The room is quiet except for the crunching of popcorn, our breathing and the movie's tense soundtrack. It's also dark: only one lamp on the end table next to us on to accompany the cold glow of the TV. Reggie has his hand resting on my thigh and every time something scary happens he grips on to it. Daniel has his arm on the back of the sofa, resting it just behind my shoulders – he keeps bringing it down around me protectively, his bare arm brushing against my neck as he does so. I can't tell if it's the film or their frequent touch on sensitive places, but my arms keep erupting in goosebumps.

I look between the two of them. Both of their faces are entranced by the film's storyline, the white TV light flickering off their skin. Reggie notices me watching him. He leans closer, his breath salty from the popcorn.

'Too scary for you, huh?' he says with a wink.

'No, it's fine!' I say.

'Sure, sure.' He chuckles and raises his eyebrows at Daniel. They both laugh and Daniel brings his arm properly around my shoulders and squeezes me in tight to him. I register the warmth of his chest through his T-shirt, the softness of his fingers on my arm. I feel my cheeks getting hot. Why is their attention feeling so different today? Is it because I want it to?

I push Daniel playfully and we all turn our faces back to the TV. The tension from the movie settles in once more . . . with something else on top. With Daniel's arm still wrapped around me, and Reggie's hand on my leg, it's as if I can feel all three of our heartbeats, pulsing gently together – except mine's beating in my pants. Am I the only one feeling curious about what's going on here?

At the next scary scene, I take the opportunity to grip on to both of their legs, squeezing my fingers into their thighs. They both mirror back a squeeze where their respective hands are resting on me, and it's not like the squeezes before. These are sensual, long, wanting squeezes. It sparks some more heat inside me. My breathing deepens; I can hear theirs doing the same.

Heartbeat thumping now, I don't move my hands off their legs. Instead, I start to massage my fingers back and forth. When neither of them stops me, I brave looking over at Daniel, searching his face for a signal that it isn't just me feeling this way. In answer, he leans closer so we're almost nose to nose, his eyes glinting hopefully in the TV's glow.

Reggie's hand strokes down the middle of my thigh, sending warm sensations rippling through me. I look over to him and feel Daniel's lips hover on my neck as I do so, causing the hairs there to stand on end. Just as Daniel kisses my neck, Reggie leans and kisses my mouth. My body is flooded with a new desire I never knew I had.

Daniel snatches my face from Reggie and kisses me too, while

Reggie's hands start wandering searchingly over my breasts and thighs. Daniel's tongue is in my mouth. I run my hands over their crotches and feel them both getting hard. It's hard to know which sensation to focus on – instead, I lean into all of them.

Without stopping to think what's happening, I let them both begin to pull at my clothes. Together they lift my T-shirt off and my breasts bounce out as the material moves past them.

Daniel's mouth drops open as he takes me in, naked in front of him for the first time. His hands move to cup me and he starts to massage my breasts and nipples. My head rushes. At the same time, Reggie pulls my joggers off my legs. He gets off the sofa and moves down to sit in front of me, between my legs, pushing them wide apart. Daniel's mouth replaces his hands on my nipples. I throw my head back and gasp as Reggie licks my pussy over the material, two mouths on me at the same time. My senses feel overwhelmed – Daniel's lips hungry and hard, while Reggie moves slowly and passionately. I feel my knickers being pushed aside. Reggie pauses for a moment and I watch him look intently at my pussy. I never knew how hot it could feel to have somebody stare at it. Reggie traces a finger over my lips, teasing me and almost as if he's noticed, Daniel does the same thing with my nipples – tracing his fingers around them, pinching and then stopping, pinching and then stopping.

Reggie pulls my knickers off and Daniel takes it as his cue to stand and pull off his T-shirt, then everything else, so that he's standing there with his hard cock in his hand. I bite my lip, watching him almost jealously tug at his own hard shaft.

As I watch Daniel, Reggie plunges his finger into my wetness, making me moan. The feeling of something inside me makes me desperate for more. He starts kissing my clit, taking his tongue in loops around me. It feels fucking amazing. He slips another finger inside as he sucks my clit. I feel almost dizzy with pleasure.

Daniel climbs on to the sofa and brings his cock close to my face. I take him into my wet mouth, wrap my tongue around it, tease the head before taking in the whole of him, down to the bottom of the shaft. Knowing that Daniel is feeling a similar pleasure to what I'm feeling between my own legs is crazy hot. After a few moments of Reggie sucking on me and me sucking on Daniel, Reggie gets up from between my legs and gets undressed too. Daniel takes his cock out of my mouth and starts lying down on the sofa. I move so that I'm sitting on top of him, his cock resting between my legs ready to pass my entrance. Reggie slots into the space between Daniel's legs behind me and strokes my back with the tips of his fingers, sending shivers down my spine. I'm ready to feel more. I push my hand between my legs and slip Daniel into me. We both gasp at the same time, whimpering in pleasure. I lean over Daniel so that our bodies are parallel to each other and Reggie's hands reach around the sides of me to squeeze my breasts and pinch my nipples. The feeling of Daniel's cock inside me filling me up at the same time as the sweet pain of the pinches is incredible.

As we all move together, a mess of tangled limbs, I feel Reggie's cock slipping between my ass cheeks in the fluids I've created. My heart races as I know what is going to happen next. His hands disappear from my breasts, squeeze my butt cheeks and then his fingers start to play with my butthole, easing in and out, relaxing me, bringing up all the wetness from my pussy. I can feel myself throbbing around Daniel, fluttering in anticipation. I kiss him deeply on the mouth, then pull away so I can look into his eyes just as Reggie pushes himself into my ass. I'm immediately plummeted into ecstasy between two men with two cocks inside me. Reggie moves slowly behind as Daniel thrusts from underneath. I reach a new dimension, pleasure rocketing through me in electrifying shocks.

'I'm going to cum,' I moan deeply.

'Yes, cum for us,' Daniel breathes into my ear.

They both thrust deeper, the rhythm intensifying and I completely lose myself.

Waves of orgasm rush through me, the pleasure too much to bear. The boys moan in appreciation as I tighten around them, throbbing on their cocks.

I collapse on to Daniel and we all lay there in a wet mess, still entangled, our breathing heavy and deep and satisfied, recovering from the intense pleasure we've just created.

In front of us, the credits roll on the TV screen.

TIP 22:

EXTERNAL AIDS

Sometimes the imagination just isn't cutting it, or you've had enough of replaying sex with your ex in your head! External aids can be amazing for leaning into your fantasies and getting new ideas to stimulate your own body. I mean, that's why I wrote this book! If you get to a point where you've used all the stories in here, or if you just want to mix it up a bit, then don't forget that other external aids exist too.

PORN

While porn can seem a bit scary to some, there is so much out there that it's hard not to find something that suits you. Try looking into feminist porn instead of the usual free websites. It's so important that we support ethically made content, so that there continues to be porn out there that's actually really educational and enjoyable to watch! Check out XConfessions for beautiful erotic cinema or Lustery for amateur homemade videos by real couples.

AUDIO PORN

If looking at other people's bodies isn't for you, then check out audio porn. You can, of course, tune into the audio version of this book to indulge your senses, but there's also plenty of audio porn subscriptions out there, such as Dipsea.

STOCKHOLM VAMPIRE

READING TIME
>10 MINUTES

THE SEXUAL PARTNER IS
CRUEL

SEXY CHECKLIST
☐ MASTURBATION
■ CLIT PLAY/FINGERING
☐ CUNNILINGUS
☐ BLOW JOB
■ NIPPLE PLAY
■ VAGINAL PENETRATION
☐ ANAL/BUTT PLAY
☐ SPANKING
☐ SEX TOYS
☐ CHOKING
■ BDSM

My eyes adjust to the room, sore from a slumber I didn't put myself in. A damp smell fills my nostrils as my eyes start to flick around me. I'm in a strange, dark room that has damp slippery walls that I can feel against my back. There's a constant dripping sound in the corner and a greenish tinge everywhere – as if I'm underwater. My arms are strapped above my head. I look up to see I'm cuffed to a wall. I try to pull my wrists free but to no avail – terror starts to flood through me. How did I get here?

I vaguely remember I was walking home from seeing friends. I only live down the road from them, so as usual, I walked back by myself. I remember the moon shining full in the sky, stars sprinkling the dark blue. Then, as I passed an alleyway, there was a strange breeze on my hair, as if something had moved very fast by me. And then: nothing. Darkness.

My heart is beating hard against my ribs. Should I scream for help? Would someone come running? Or would it make whoever brought me here aware that I'm awake? I look around desperately for an escape. All the corners of the room are very dark, but I spot an open door to a corridor where the light is even greener. As I hone in on it, a piercing scream echoes from whatever lies beyond it. My skin prickles with goosebumps, my forehead beading with sweat. I close my eyes and squeeze, hoping to wake up from a nightmare.

When I open them, there is a dark figure standing in the doorway. I go to scream but my fear traps my voice in my throat. The figure moves across the room as if it were floating, and yet I can see its feet touching the ground. It stops in a shadow across the other side of the room and I swear all I can see are two red eyes. My whole body is trembling, my feet almost losing balance on the wet floor.

The figure breathes in a sharp intake of air as if it's tasting it. Then a long sigh of pleasure emanates from the corner.

'Who are you?' I try to shout, but find my word is a whisper instead.

The figure floats forward out of the shadows. 'Shouldn't you ask: *what* am I?' A flash of white fangs. Can it be? No. I'm dreaming. Or this is a sick joke. They don't exist in real life.

In a flash he's next to me where I can't quite see him. 'Take a guess,' he says quietly into my ear. It's strange: he's so close to me and yet I can't feel any breath on me. All I can feel is my own breath, short and shallow in my chest.

He moves around to face me. He smells intoxicating, of all my favourite things in the world. He's deathly pale and sharply handsome; his eyes are indeed red, and his fangs, his fangs . . .

'Vampire,' I whisper.

He laughs gleefully. 'Very good,' he says. He sniffs the air again, sighs again.

'Why are you doing that?' I whimper.

He smiles with his beautiful mouth, his fangs bared once more. 'Because you smell oh so delicious,' he says.

'Please, let me go,' I beg, pulling on my chains so that they clank together. 'I'll do anything.'

He watches me writhe and then says, 'I can see you're getting distressed. I'll leave you to get some rest.'

He glides towards the door and I don't know whether to be relieved that he's leaving so soon or terrified that I'll be alone again. But before I can think anything else, I'm asleep once more.

I wake to find . . . I'm in a bathroom. This time lying against the moist, hard stones of the floor. He must have moved me while I was under his influenced sleep. There's a roll-top bathtub in the middle of the room. Curiously I sit up and peer in, half expecting it to be full of blood. It's a huge tub and the water is running, steam billowing off it, and I can see bubbles and rose petals on the rising surface. The smell of the products drifts towards me – sweet and magical. I look around, having no clue what's going on, when shivers dance down my body.

He's back. The vampire.

'Would you like to get in?' he says from the shadowy doorway, his voice soft and melting.

I swallow and look back at the hot water. It looks mesmerising. I do actually want nothing more than to wash the damp slime off my skin. 'If I do, will you be in here?' I ask.

He comes forward into the green light. 'Naturally,' he says with a flash of his fangs.

I feel disgusting from the room I've been chained up in. The bath looks so inviting . . .

I nod. The vampire offers me a hand, and in a blink I'm on my feet. I walk unsteadily towards the bath.

'Will you turn around while I undress?' I ask him.

To my surprise he turns. I start to undo my slime-covered blouse –

dropping it to the floor, taking my humbling human speed to remove everything until I'm standing there naked. I look quickly over at him, to see if he's looked at my body, but he's still facing the other way. I step quickly into the hot water, eager to not be exposed near him.

As soon as I'm in, I feel my whole body relax. It's not like water I've ever felt on my skin before. It's like bathing in silk or velvet. I sink my body beneath it, the bubbles covering me up.

The vampire turns around. In one swift movement he's beside the bathtub. He turns off the tap, and tells me he needs to chain my wrists to its sides. I don't have much choice.

As he takes my first wrist, I notice that the contrast of his freezing fingers on my skin, which is hot from the water, feels incandescent. When he takes my second wrist, his fingers pause on the throbbing pulse in my veins. I look quickly up at him, alarmed at the flashing of his red eyes. But once my wrist is secure, he lets go of me. I'm finding this situation more tantalising than I should: the fear of knowing what he is, that I'm his prisoner, is mixing with my undeniable attraction towards him. As he leans away, he takes his intoxicating smell with him and disappointment surges through me.

He moves to the end of the bath and takes off his crisp suit jacket. For a second, I think he might be about to get into the bath and a perverse thrill shoots through me. But then I realise he's not undressing – he's rolling up the sleeves of his shirt. 'As you are . . . incapacitated,' he says, 'can I help you wash yourself?'

I should say no. I should want to run a mile from here. But I want to know what it feels like to be washed by a vampire.

I nod once more.

He grabs a sponge from behind the taps. He dips it into the water, beginning with my feet. He uses one hand to wash, the other to hold me steady. Once again, the coldness of his body mixed with the heat of the water is sensational; it begins to send vibrations through me.

When he gets to the top of my thighs, he skips over my pussy and gets to work on my stomach, tenderly stroking it and rubbing it with the slightly rough sponge. A strange feeling trickles through me; I think I might be hoping he'll wash my breasts next . . . but again he skips them, going instead to the top of my chest before he begins to wipe down my arms. All the while, my eyes follow his handsome, whiter-than-snow face.

Now he looks at me. 'I shall free your arms so you may wash the rest,' he says.

'No,' I say quickly, almost by accident. 'I don't mind.'

He surveys me with his red eyes. 'I shall only do it if you ask me,' he says.

'Please,' I hear myself say. 'Please wash me.'

As soon as the words are out of my mouth, he smiles cruelly and I think: *He's planned this. He knew he could make me want more.* But it doesn't change the fact that I do.

His hand slips back into the bathwater. The sponge slowly circles one nipple and then the other. And then he drags it down my body to my pussy. I open my legs and he rubs the sponge over it. The friction on my clit makes me almost cry out. I wish he'd swap the sponge for his hand. I want to have the feel of his cold finger push against my lips.

My eyes are on his arm disappearing into the water between my legs, but I can feel that his eyes are on me. 'You have only to ask,' he whispers.

I take a deep breath. 'Please,' I say.

'Please what?' he says, with another cruel smile.

'Fuck me,' I say.

In a blink I'm out of the bath; he has uncuffed me and scooped me up into his arms at lightning speed. Before I have time even to think, we're back in the other dungeon and he is cuffing my hands back to the wall above me. The water from the bath drips down my body as he undresses before me with such speed that he is suddenly naked. I stare, mouth open, at his big, hard, stiff cock. He moves towards me and I feel it, cold as ice, caress my pussy.

I lean into him and kiss his cold hard lips; they send a shiver through me. He tastes exactly how he smells: it's intoxicating. He hungrily kisses me back, slipping his cool wet tongue into my mouth.

The sexual tension is strangling my fear – the mixture of both is extremely exciting. He races his hands over my naked flesh at a speed that sends shockwaves into my pussy. I purposely pull at my chains, the excitement of being his prisoner fuelling my pleasure. His cool mouth descends onto my nipples and he grazes me with his fangs – as he sucks, my nipples harden in his mouth. My moans echo over the stone walls.

He teases his cold cock against my warm entrance. I gasp at the sensation against me, wetness immediately pooling, dripping down him. He leans in to kiss my neck, my pulse visibly drumming against my skin under his lips – fear flickers through me before he plunges himself inside. His stone-hard cock fills me up. Fuck. My cuffs rattle against the wall as he thrusts deeper. My warm breasts press against his cold chest. My breathing becomes heavy as he plunges, and he reaches around me to claw his fingers into my butt cheeks. Moans ripple out from my throat as I bury my face into his neck, sniffing him in as he does the same to me.

He's getting closer and closer and I want him to fill me up with his icy vampire cum. I feel my own pleasure rise as I look into his red eyes, as he runs his fingernails down my outstretched arms, from the back of my elbows, down over my armpits and down to my nipples. He's getting closer and closer, and my own pleasure is edging towards climax too. I bite down hard on my lip to edge around my orgasm.

My pussy tightens around him one last time – and then I give in to my pleasure, letting my muscles spasm, allowing the chains above me to bear my weight. He holds me up by my ass to keep me steady as he thrusts once more and cums inside me. I've never felt more alive, the blood pumps through my veins and . . . I can taste some on my lip, from where I bit myself just now. I lick it away, but he's caught the smell of it.

His eyes widen at the sight of it pooling where I've cut myself. There is nothing I can do but let him lean forward and lick the area where it's forming. I breathe heavily, waiting to see what happens next.

He bares his fangs.

CERVIX PLEASURE

Cervix pleasure does exist! Not everyone feels sensations in the deep dark depths of their vaginas, but some definitely do, so if you're comfortable with the idea, it's worth a good go finding out if you're in their camp. Here's how to try:

STEP 1: Make sure you know where your cervix is. It is inside your vagina, towards the back and up. (Google a diagram to get the clearest idea.)

STEP 2: You're going to need a toy you can penetrate yourself with. Lube it up.

STEP 3: Either (or you can do both!): Pulse the toy against the cervix with an in/out motion or circle the toy against the cervix with a rocking motion

STEP 4: As you do this, breathe deeply into the sensations to allow yourself to register these new feelings.

The cervix pleasure will probably feel different to you than clitoral or G-spot pleasure. If clitoral orgasms feel like a firework, G-spot like fire, then a cervical orgasm would be like an electric current radiating deep inside. I'd definitely recommend adding clitoral stimulation for max pleasure!

WHEN GOOD NEIGHBOURS BECOME GOOD FRIENDS

READING TIME

>10 MINUTES

THE SEXUAL PARTNERS ARE

MANY

SEXY CHECKLIST

☐ MASTURBATION
■ CLIT PLAY/FINGERING
■ CUNNILINGUS
■ BLOW JOB
■ NIPPLE PLAY
■ VAGINAL PENETRATION
☐ ANAL/BUTT PLAY
■ SPANKING
☐ SEX TOYS
☐ CHOKING
■ BDSM

My new address is Flat C, Cornucopia House. Flats A and B are on the
floor below me and both belong to married couples; Flat A – Emmanuel
and Erica – seem a little aloof, while Flat B – Andrew and Amelia –
are very friendly. The other flat on my own floor belongs to a woman
with headmistress vibes, who I only know as Ms Hunter because I've
forgotten her first name and that's how her post is addressed.

It's Saturday night and I find myself nervously knocking on the
door of Flat B. Andrew and Amelia both open it to invite me in.
Andrew kisses my cheek and praises me on my wine choice; Amelia
wraps her arms around me as if she's known me for ages. In truth, we
only met for five minutes in the hallway yesterday, which is when she
asked me to this dinner party. I've been stressed with the move and so
I lean into the hug more than I probably would normally. She smells
of good cooking and perfume.

Emmanuel and Erica are sitting on the sofa in the open-plan
kitchen–living room, looking bored. Ms Hunter is standing over
them both and complaining about next door, who leave out food for
foxes. It means in the middle of the night she's woken by the sounds of
them having vociferous sex.

Andrew hands out large glasses of wine and everyone sits around
the table. They all put their attention on me, asking me questions
about where I've moved from, what I do, what my hobbies are. Having
five strangers stare at you for a long time – and they're all unusually
good at eye contact – feels oddly satisfying and intimidating at the
same time. I'm glad of the wine in my hand.

For dessert, Andrew has made chocolate fondant. I've noticed that Emmanuel and Erica are very tactile with each other. All night they've been stroking the back of each other's necks, or giving each other's hands a squeeze. Now Emmanuel gets chocolate on the corner of his mouth and Erica leans forward to lick it off. She notices my eyes on her from across the table as she does this. Without breaking eye contact with me, she kisses Emmanuel full on the lips, slipping her tongue in for good measure. I look away quickly, and Erica laughs.

It's after dinner that things really begin to change. Ms Hunter suggests we play a game of 'Most likely to'. We each have to say something like 'forget bin day'. Then at the count of three, we all point at the person we think is most likely to do it. Whoever gets the most fingers pointed at them has to do a forfeit.

Andrew is the first to make the questions 'adult'. As he pours out more wine, he says, 'Most likely to be a dark horse in bed.' Everyone points at Ms Hunter. The questions get dirtier from there, but the forfeits stay clean until Amelia asks, 'Most likely to receive a blow job in the hallway.' All fingers point at Emmanuel and we all laugh, the wine making us giddy, the sexual nature of the questions making us alert.

Andrew jokes that as a forfeit, Emmanuel should go into the hallway and get that blow job – and then Erica stands up and holds her hand out to Emmanuel. She leads him out to the corridor while we go quiet, grinning at each other; surely they're just joking? Surely Erica can't actually be down on her knees out there? 'I'm going to go look through the peephole,' Amelia giggles.

Just as she gets up, the lights go off. The clocks on the oven and microwave have disappeared too. Ms Hunter says she'll look out of the window and we hear her shuffling to the curtains. No lights are on in the street either. It's a power cut. The atmosphere in the room ironically gets even more electric.

The front door opens and Erica and Emmanuel come back in, making a joke (is it a joke?) about their fun being interrupted, while Andrew and Amelia start lighting the candles on the mantelpiece. The glow they create is much dimmer than a lamp, and sensual shadows fall over everyone's faces. Ms Hunter starts telling us a story about a power cut when she was a teenager, when she played spin the bottle with her friends – should we do it now? Amelia squeals with glee and goes to find one of our empties. I look around to see if anyone will say they don't want to. As mad as it sounds considering I don't know these people, the suggestion has made me excited. I'm feeling warm from the wine and tingly from the game we've just played. A kiss would be just the thing to round off the evening.

We sit in a circle on the floor, in the space between the three sofas which surround the fireplace. The wine bottle is placed in the middle. I look around at everybody's candlelit faces and feel butterflies in my stomach.

Andrew goes first. He gets Emmanuel. They crawl towards each other and it's as if everyone takes a breath. Their kiss isn't long . . . but it's not short either.

Emmanuel spins next and gets Erica. The breath everyone was holding streams out in an angry laugh at such a cop-out given the two of them are married. After Erica and Emmanuel have given each other an affectionate peck, Erica spins.

The bottle twists so quickly it's hard to keep your eye on it. Then eventually it begins to slow down . . . on to me. Erica is sitting next to me. She turns her face to mine. Before she leans in, she brushes the hair off my face. Then she kisses me. Her mouth feels soft and warm on mine. She pulls away and says, 'You're so tense. It's just a game.'

I would think Erica doesn't like me very much, except she now gets on her knees behind my back and starts to massage my neck with her hands. She's still touching me while I lean down to spin the bottle. It lands on Emmanuel. He comes towards me and kisses me deeply on the mouth, while Erica continues to knead the base of my neck with her fingers. Both sensations together feel intense, sending a thrill of goosebumps over my skin.

Emmanuel pulls away. 'I like this new game,' Ms Hunter says matter-of-factly. She tells Emmanuel to kiss me again, and this time for Amelia to get behind him and give him a massage. Andrew asks her what he should do. Ms Hunter thinks about it and then says, 'Massage Erica's breasts.'

Andrew looks at Erica and she smiles and nods. I watch with my mouth open as she pulls her top up to her bra, and pulls the cups down so her breasts and nipples are exposed over the top. Andrew sits behind her so that the base of her bum is in his crotch, and then takes his fingertips to her breasts and starts to massage them with his palms and his fingertips. Watching this happen is so erotic that I feel my pussy throb.

Emmanuel puts his finger under my chin and turns me back to face him. Behind him I can see Amelia stroking her fingers down the back of his neck. He looks at me for permission and, when I nod, he puts his tongue back in my mouth and I close my eyes as we swirl them around. He still tastes of chocolate and his tongue is hot, wet and nimble.

When we pull apart, we instinctively turn to Ms Hunter for our next instructions. She looks thoughtful again, then tells Amelia and Erica to undress each other, and for Andrew and Emmanuel to do the same. I don't know whether to look at Amelia as Erica pulls her dress off and reveals her standing there in just her knickers, or to look at Andrew as he gets on his knees and undoes the button and zip on Emmanuel's jeans, roughly pulling down on the belt loops to reveal Emmanuel's briefs with a boner inside them.

Gradually, four sets of clothes come off, and in front of me, glowing in the candlelight, are two sets of breasts with erect nipples, two hard cocks pointing to the ceiling and two naked pussies. I watch on hungrily as the two couples look each other over appraisingly.

'What about her?' Erica asks Ms Hunter, pointing at me.
'You can *all* undress her,' Ms Hunter says.

My heart begins to pound in my ears. Adrenalin seeps through my insides, turning me on.

Four warm hands pull me up from where I've been sitting cross-legged on the floor. Erica and Emmanuel stand behind me and Andrew and Amelia stand in front. Erica and Amelia pull my top up, their fingers tickling my stomach as they take it off, while Andrew and Emmanuel pull my skirt down so that I'm standing in my underwear, their hot breath on my back and the base of my stomach. Erica pulls the straps of my bra tightly together to undo the clasp, and then Amelia runs her fingers down my arms as she pulls off the straps. Meanwhile, Emmanuel and Andrew take one side of my pants each and stroke them down my legs. The sensation of having four sets of hands on you at the same time is like nothing I've ever felt before. My heartbeat flutters with a nervous excitement as I stand before them all, completely naked.

Amelia takes my hands and puts them on her breasts, a smile flickering at the corner of her lips. I feel the soft squishiness of them wondrously with my fingers. A sharp jolt of pain pleasingly snaps me back into my own body. I look down – Ms Hunter is squeezing my nipple sharply.

She looks around at all of us.

'The rules of the game are that you are only allowed to do what I tell you. Is that understood?'

I find myself nodding eagerly. I can't believe the situation I've found myself in – or how wet I am because of it. My clit seems to be spasming without anybody having even touched it. We all turn to Ms Hunter obediently, waiting to be told our next moves.

She tells us to sit in a circle so that clockwise, we are Amelia, Erica, Andrew, me and Emmanuel. She wants us to play 'oral pass the parcel' where we will all take it in turns to use our mouths on the next person's genitals for thirty seconds while the others watch. My eyes are wide as I watch Erica spread her legs so Amelia can put her mouth to her pussy; I am jealous of the tongue that is running over Erica's clit and the look on her face at the pleasure it's releasing in her. I want it to be my turn.

But first I will watch Erica deepthroat Andrew's cock into her mouth, see the saliva dribble down his thick shaft as she pulls up and down on it. Now Erica is pulling her mouth off him and using her hand to stimulate him further; she's made his cock so wet her hand slips and slides around him. Ms Hunter sharply tells her to stand up. We all hold our breaths, not knowing what's going to happen next.

Ms Hunter tells Erica she broke the rules – the rules are we can only use our mouths, not our hands. She makes Erica go over to the sofa and bend over the arm and then she spanks her, three loud, hard claps on each cheek. My pussy throbs even more. I exchange a giddy glance with Emmanuel, who seems to be almost salivating.

As Erica sits back down, I realise it's my turn. I bend my legs at the knees and open them wide, lean back on to my elbows. From between my legs, Andrew smiles mischievously at me. And then he puts his mouth to my clit. The warmth it elicits in me is incredible. His tongue feels sensational on my clit. He laps between my pussy lips with abandon, then back up to focus on my clit.

Emmanuel asks Ms Hunter if we can 'modify' the rules. Can the rest join in . . . at the same time? Ms Hunter pauses to think, and then says we can, except for Erica, because she still needs to learn her lesson. She really is living up to the 'headmistress' moniker I've given her. Erica pouts back at her.

Emmanuel grabs a cushion from the sofa and pushes it under my head. Then he kneels either side of my face so that his cock is right in front of my mouth. Amelia stands with her foot either side of my head, facing Emmanuel. First Emmanuel eases his cock into my mouth. The feel of his hard shaft filling me up while Andrew laps on my clitoris is almost too much. But when I look up and see that Emmanuel is also sucking on Amelia's clit, I want to explode.

A loud strict voice interrupts us: Ms Hunter telling us to stop what we're doing. The anticipation of not knowing what's going to happen next is erotic as hell.

She tells us to all stand up in a line, and then she paces in front of all of us like a drill master, looking at each of our naked bodies in turn. The candlelight makes her appear even more fierce than before. She runs her hand up and down Andrew's erect cock. She puts two fingers in Amelia's mouth and tells her to suck on them. Then she gets to me. I take a deep breath in and a deep breath out. She looks down at my pussy, gets on her knees and runs her thumb from my wet clit down to my wet pussy and pushes in. I gasp at the pleasure of it.

She tells me to lie on my side on the floor. As I'm doing as I'm told, she walks up and down the line again. She stops in front of Emmanuel. I'm desperate for her to tell him to come and fuck me and she seems to know this because she looks at me while she draws the suspense out. Finally, she gives me what I want. She tells him to get down behind me and put his cock in me.

The warmth of Emmanuel's stomach as he spoons me and the feel of his hard cock on my back are incredible. He asks me if this is okay. I need something inside me so badly I find myself begging him to do it. As he pushes his cock into my wetness, I close my eyes and let out a deep, guttural moan.

When I open my eyes, Amelia is in front of me, her breasts pooling to one side. She still smells of good cooking and perfume. Spooning her is Erica, and spooning Erica is Andrew. Andrew has started fucking Erica and she's moaning too.

Ms Hunter tells Erica to fuck Amelia with her fingers, and tells Amelia to rub my clit. Having Emmanuel thrust into me from behind and Amelia's warm fingers slipping over my clitoris is heavenly and I feel my climax start to build. I look down and see Amelia's leg slightly raised, allowing Erica to dive two fingers into her pussy. The look of pure joy on Amelia's face makes me want to kiss her. I ask Ms Hunter if I'm allowed but she says no, her eyes flickering mischievously with power.

I can't kiss her, but fuck it, I want to touch her. I ask Amelia if I can touch her clit and she says yes enthusiastically. I reach my hand down and begin to rub her and she cries out with the pleasure of it. She feels so soft and wet and warm under my hand.

But Ms Hunter has seen. She tells Emmanuel to fuck me harder in punishment and she leans down and pinches my nipple again. It's all too much: the feeling of Emmanuel's hard cock pulsing inside me, the sensations in my clitoris as Amelia's fingers slip over it, the sound of Erica's moans as Andrew fucks her, the feel of Amelia's soft, engorged pussy under my hands and now the flash of pain in my nipple. **I lean back into Emmanuel and I cum so hard and so loudly that I'm glad all my neighbours are here in this room so that there's no one to hear me.**

Amelia pushes her naked body against me as I tremble to stillness, Emmanuel holding me close to him comfortingly.

Into my ear she whispers, 'We do this every Saturday night.'

TIP 24:

SQUIRTING

Is female ejaculation a myth for porn or is it real? And if it is real, is it 'wetness' or is it just piss? I'm going to boldly assert that we've all wondered about it at one time or another. There's no conclusive answers to these questions (research on the female body is still ludicrously poor), but all we really need to know is that, however you define what's actually going on, some vulvas squirt every time they have sex, others maybe occasionally and some never!

In case you have a burning desire to make it happen – I'm a big believer in giving everything a go at least once – I'm going to give you my advice so you can maybe try it out during the next story. For the record, I've had a plethora of men between my legs trying to do it for me and I think only one managed to get a little puddle. The things they did might have worked on others, but not me – like everything in this book, it takes exploration and discovery to see what your body responds to. That said, let me tell you what worked for me and then you can give it a go if you want to!

STEP 1: Seems obvious but you do need to be pretty hydrated.

STEP 2: Prepare by laying down a towel or being somewhere you don't mind getting wet! This is so you don't have to worry about soaking your mattress while you try it out! As we talked about on page 22, worrying can be a big turn off.

STEP 3: Find your most relaxed state with some deep breaths and focus on your pleasure (you could try the simple breathing technique on page 57.

STEP 4: Insert a toy (or your fingers) in a way that hits your G-spot area. Repeat the movement in a 'come hither' motion.

STEP 5 : With your free hand, press on the mound of your pubic region, just below your stomach and above your vulva.

STEP 6: Instead of clenching your muscles in pleasure, you want to relax them, maybe even push a little.

STEP 7: Continuously rock in the pleasure zone with a firmer pressure and higher speed.

STEP 8: If you feel the need to pee, that's the squirt, so don't hold back!

STEP 9: Fully let go and don't stop with the motion.

NOTE: Sometimes squirting can link up with your orgasm, other times it might happen before – this is totally normal!

PEGGING

READING TIME
<7 MINUTES

THE SEXUAL PARTNER IS
SUBMISSIVE

SEXY CHECKLIST
☐ MASTURBATION
☐ CLIT PLAY/FINGERING
■ CUNNILINGUS
☐ BLOW JOB
☐ NIPPLE PLAY
☐ VAGINAL PENETRATION
■ ANAL/BUTT PLAY
☐ SPANKING
■ SEX TOYS
☐ CHOKING
■ BDSM

A week ago, my boyfriend asked me if we could watch porn together and touch ourselves. Recently our sex has been getting a little samey, so I gladly agreed. We chose a video each. In his choice, a woman wearing black shiny latex with a mask over her eyes took a man into a dungeon, told him to strip and then she donned a strap-on. I'd never have picked it, but it was hot. The role reversal was immensely erotic.

After we'd both cum, when we were brushing our teeth getting ready for bed, I could see my boyfriend working himself up to say something: he kept tensing his shoulders, taking a breath and then swallowing and looking away. I knew what it was he wanted to ask. I thought about what I'd say if he did. It would definitely be a new experience, and watching porn with him had shown me I was craving novelty. We didn't own any toys that stimulated his prostate – I liked the idea of being the one to give him that sort of pleasure for the first time. And the thought of standing behind him, fucking him the way he fucked me, feeling like a man with the power to penetrate, turned me on. I took my toothbrush out of my mouth and put him out of his misery: 'If you want to try pegging, I'm game.'

All this week we've been working up to it. Each night, he's lain down naked on the bed and I've sat fully clothed behind him in the space between his legs. I've squeezed lube over a butt plug, circled it around his asshole and then gently pushed it in. Even this small taste of power has thrilled me. The butt plugs have got a little bigger as the week's gone on, testing out his thresholds. Some nights I've pushed one into him before dinner and made him sit there with it in, spooling spaghetti around my fork and watching him, aroused, at the table. Other nights

I've massaged his back and then his butt cheeks, spreading them wide so I could see the base of the plug looking up at me.

And now tonight is the night. I've bought the harness and strap-on. He's done all the prep work he can. We're ready to go.

In the bathroom, I tie my hair up and take off my top and bra, but leave my jeans on. I've told him to wait in the bedroom for me naked. When I turn the door handle, he's sitting on the edge of the bed next to the harness and dildo I've laid out, gripping the curve of the mattress nervously. I walk over to him and kiss him; a very deep kiss, my tongue filling the whole of his mouth. I take off my jeans and knickers and tell him to put them away like a good boy. My pussy tingles as he does what I say.

I tell him to get on his knees by my feet and to kiss them while I prepare to fuck him. The sensation of him doing this tickles in a way that I can feel in my pussy.

Strap-on securely fastened, I look down at him by my feet and tell him to suck it. 'I want you to make it really wet and ready for your ass,' I say.

He does as he's told. Watching him deepthroat the dildo sends a rush of adrenalin through me. The power in this new dynamic is setting me on fire.

'You're doing really well,' I tell him. Saliva drips down the shaft of the dildo and dribbles on to my naked pussy underneath. I put my hands in his hair so that I can feel his head bob up and down. He looks up at me longingly as he sucks and I feel my pussy burn.

I tell him to get on the bed. He does, taking up a position on all fours.

I stand next to the bed right behind him. There's a mirror over our chest of drawers directly to the left of us. I look at us: a magnificent picture – me totally naked with a big hard cock erect before me, him on all fours in front of me, also with a big, hard cock dangling between his legs. I look back at what's in front of me. He's sticking his ass up slightly, desperate for my touch. I suck my finger, coating it with as much saliva as possible, and push it inside his asshole, moving in and out gently. It feels warm and oh so tight around my finger. I notice the pleasure he's feeling by the way his body moves back towards me. My own pussy flutters beneath my strap-on at his excitement. I could do it now, could plunge the dildo into him, but I'm enjoying my power too much.

I tell him to turn over so he's lying on his back. I move on to the bed and straddle his face, then tell him to open his mouth. He does. 'I think you need to do a better job with this,' I say. I push the dildo down and fill his mouth up again. He grabs on to my ass, trying to control the situation, but I remove his arms and pin them above his head. I continue to fuck his mouth. We look into each other's eyes. He's loving this, and I'm loving it too.

He takes his mouth off the dildo. I tell him it's harder than it looks, isn't it?

I tell him to get back on all fours. On my way back to his ass, I grab the lube. I squeeze the bottle above his butt crack so that it runs in between his cheeks. He trembles at the coldness of it. I use my warm hand to move it around over his asshole and he trembles some more. I plunge two fingers in this time and he moans.

'I'm going to put my cock inside you now,' I tell him. I feel so powerful. My nipples are hard with desire, I know my pussy is engorged, and yet the cock between my legs feels like it belongs to me.

I take the dildo in one hand and rub it against his wet hole. He moans greedily, wanting it more than ever. A rush of adrenalin pumps through me as I comprehend what I'm about to do. I'm about to fuck my boyfriend in a way I never thought I would. Pleasure surges through me.

I push the dildo into his lubed-up ass slowly, inch by inch. He gasps below me and then breathes in and out deeply.

'Tell me how it feels,' I command him.

'So . . . good,' is all he can manage.

I push deeper inside him and his body crumples back into me as he rocks against me in pleasure. I look in the mirror again at myself, at how incredible I look pulling out of him and pushing back in. At how much I love that he's on all fours, taking it like I normally take it.

'I'm so fucking deep in your ass,' I say, turning myself on with this new power craze I'm riding, pushing back and forth, thrusting into him. His moans are provoking my movements, his pleasure making my clit pulse without me even touching it. 'Tell me how it feels to be fucked.'

'It feels . . . full,' he gasps as I push deeper. My cock fills him up completely and rocks on his prostate. I can see from the mirror that he looks like he's on another planet – another planet of pleasure. 'It feels . . . hard.'

'Yes,' I say, leaning over him and running my fingernails from his neck down to the base of his back.

He moans again at this extra sensation. 'It feels so good to have you inside me,' he breathes.

'I love being inside you,' I say. Pleasure is rocketing through me. 'You're doing so well taking my cock.' I reach around him and take his own cock in my hand. An animalistic sound ruptures from his throat. His body squirms under me. I stroke his cock and push myself deeper inside him. I smack his butt cheek and tell him, 'You're such a *good* boy.'

His body convulses and his cock pulses in my hand, shooting his cum down on to the sheets. He falls down flat with the longest moan I've ever heard come out of him. I look down at him satisfied, smiling at my handiwork. I pull out very gently and slowly, my pussy throbbing, and undo the strap-on. As I throw it on the floor, he rolls over and looks up at me, his chest heaving, his eyes closed, looking as if he's never been happier in his whole life. He opens his eyes and grins at me. 'Thank you,' he says.

'My pleasure,' I say, getting up off the bed. 'Now clean up all this mess.'

TIP 25:

GET THE MIRROR BACK OUT

You probably aren't reading this book chronologically, so I don't know how long ago you read 'The Top Tip' and sat with your legs spread in front of the mirror. But I'm going to now ask you to do it again.

One of the benefits of masturbation that I mentioned in the introduction is that it can make you feel better about your body. When we masturbate we want to be having sex with ourselves, in an ultimate act of self-care. And that's what this tip is all about.

Looking in the mirror can be hard for many people, let alone looking at their naked body and their vulva. But within this act there is such power, courage and bravery, which ultimately is a key to unlocking your full pleasure potential. I want you to leave this book feeling like you've connected with yourself further than you ever have before and to inspire you to feel pleasure with your full body and mind. Which is why I invite you to sit in front of a mirror, whatever you have available to you, and touch yourself. When you look at yourself, I want you to reassure yourself that self-love and solo sex is normal and fucking amazing. I want you to tell yourself how amazing you are. How beautiful you are. How magical you are. Mirror play is the ultimate solo sex, however you want to express it.

I know that this can sound daunting, I've been there too. I've been on a roller coaster with my body confidence and how I feel about looking at myself in the mirror. It's hard to appreciate your own body when we see all these Photoshopped, face-tuned images everywhere. Step one in being confident in your own skin is surrounding yourself with positive influences. Get rid of the people you follow on social media that make you feel less, and start including people that show natural bodies. I highly suggest checking out the online magazine Sunday Morning View, which celebrates all bodies and highlights the art in the things we've been taught are wrong and imperfect.

There are a few things that have helped me get to a place where I can look in the mirror and feel really fucking hot. One was doing a boudoir photoshoot. Sounds nerve-racking, right? I was shaking in my little lace undies, that's for sure. But throughout the shoot I felt more and more comfortable, I even started to enjoy myself. I became the sexy person I knew I was inside. When it came to looking at the photos, I thought to myself, *I'm not going to like any of them, I don't like photos of myself, especially if I'm trying to be sexy, let alone almost naked.* I was shocked to discover that I loved almost every single one. I started to see myself in a different way.

To continue on this discovery of my inner confidence and acceptance of my body, my bestie Reed Amber (from ComeCurious) and I created the thirty-day nude challenge. This is a challenge where you take a nude photo of yourself at different angles every single day for thirty days, just for yourself. The more you see your body, the more you see the beauty in it. I would really encourage you to give this a go.

After we finished the challenge, I felt so proud of my body that I vowed to myself: if I ever look at myself in the mirror and think, *Wow, I look hot today*, it is my duty to take a photo so I can remember that feeling on days where I'm feeling down on myself. Because like everything, these moods and feelings come in waves. There will be good days and bad days, and that's okay! Why not try it out?

Lastly, stop the negative comments on yourself. We've all been there, prodding our stomachs or thinking mean things about our appearance. It is now the time to relearn and rethink those negative thoughts and change them into positive ones. Look into the mirror and tell yourself all the things you love about your body. This might be hard at first, but persevere. I love my boobs. I love my butt. I love my stomach. I love my lips. I love my hips. Try it, the more you repeat it the more you will start to believe it.

Back to the mirror – this tip is whatever you want to make it. It might be just standing in front of the mirror and saying positive affirmations before you dig into the meditation.

MY LOVER
THE ROCK GOD

READING TIME

>10 MINUTES

THE SEXUAL PARTNER IS

SEXY AND FAMOUS

SEXY CHECKLIST

■ MASTURBATION
■ CLIT PLAY/FINGERING
□ CUNNILINGUS
■ BLOW JOB
■ NIPPLE PLAY
■ VAGINAL PENETRATION
□ ANAL/BUTT PLAY
□ SPANKING
□ SEX TOYS
□ CHOKING
□ BDSM

A mass of sweaty bodies jump around me, punching the air to the beat as his deep, buttery voice swims around the stadium. This is the fourth time I've seen him on his latest tour; last week I achieved the impossible and was pressed up against the barrier, mere feet away from him. Today I'm a few rows back, hypnotised by the way he moves around the stage. When he comes back to the microphone stand to sing, arms outstretched, his lips brush it, and because I'm so close I can clearly see the slight stubble on his chin and the way his T-shirt clings to his chest. Even though I know the lyrics off by heart, I hang on his every word, dancing with abandon as if my life depends on it.

The next song starts, and he doesn't need to sing it because we're all belting out the lyrics so loudly. He bends his knees slightly, tips his head back and laughs, amazed at our volume, and then looks out over the crowd, to the left, to the right, and then, as his eyes roam over the section of us just in front of him, they linger on me. For a second I think I'm imagining it. But as he starts singing the words, his mouth moving in sync with mine, I know it's for real – his eyes are locked with my eyes. My all-time favourite rock star hasn't just noticed me, he's *singing* to me. I've always thought he was hot, yet I'm surprised at how intensely I'm feeling the shockwaves deep, deep inside me.

I can't hold his gaze any longer because I feel so naked underneath it. By the time I work up the courage to look back he's moved stage left. Damn. I can't wait to tell Isla, though – she was supposed to come with me tonight but she's got a migraine. I remind myself that I need to buy her something from the merchandise stand on my way home to cheer her up.

I know the setlist back to front, and when the lights dim at the end of this song, the drums still playing a soft beat to keep the adrenalin of the crowd going, I know it's because he's running off one final time before re-emerging for his big finale. When the lights finally come back up, a swelling applause erupting around the stadium as they do, the girl in front of me turns around. She leans forward and shouts into my ear, 'Security wants you!' She's pointing forwards – two rows of people in front of us is the barrier. A huge muscle man dressed in black is beckoning to me. I look around, thinking he must be wanting somebody else, but no, it's me he's calling over. I push with difficulty through to the front of the crowd and he holds his hands out to me, indicating I should climb over the barrier. I don't know what I've done wrong and I want to stay for the final song, but it's too loud for me to say that so I let him put his hands under my armpits and lift me up and over.

'What's going on?' I try to shout into his ear now I'm next to him, but he takes my hand and marches me off to the side of the stage and through a door. I can still hear the music out here but it's muffled, replaced by a tell-tale ringing in my ears.

Now the man explains. Grinning over his shoulder at me, he says, 'You're going to a party.'

Heart beating fast from not knowing what this means, I'm taken to a large, windowless room that's filling up with chatting, laughing people wearing VIP and staff lanyards, who must have just watched the concert from the wings of the stage. The security man hands me over to a woman, whispering something in her ear. She grins at me, pulls me into a hug of greeting and then music – *his* music – starts blasting over the speakers into the room. I love this song so much that I don't need any encouragement to start dancing around with her. Besides, elation is running through me: I think this must be the afterparty? After all this time, am I finally going to get to meet him?

When the door to the room next opens, a cheer goes up. It must be because he's come in. My heart starts pumping at a speed it's never known before. I can't see him properly because he's being cornered by what I assume are his friends and family; I decide that when the crowd around him gets smaller, I'll make my move. No way have I made it this far to not say hello. And in the back of my mind is the small, excited thrill that this is because he saw me in the crowd. For whatever reason, he's invited me up here.

Heart rate still pelting, I start dancing again, but only make it through the chorus before someone touches my arm . . .

I turn around.

And there he is. Smiling casually, his hair damp from sweat, his T-shirt sticking to his pecs. I press my lips together, my smile widening uncontrollably across my face. Without thinking, I reach out and take his hand in mine and enthusiastically shake it. His hot palm feels like silk in mine. He looks amused that I've done this, so I explain: 'I needed to make sure you weren't a mirage.'

He laughs my comment off, as if he's embarrassed by it, and introduces himself – which is funny because obviously I know exactly who he is. I ask him if he's the reason I'm up here. 'I've seen you before at my shows,' he says. The sound of his deep voice so close to me is mad. He's even hotter now I can see the creases around his eyes and the ever so slight dimples in his cheeks. Neither of us seems able to tear our eyes off each other and I wonder what he's thinking about me. 'I love the way you dance,' he says. 'I guess I couldn't bear the thought of not seeing you dance again.'

Just when I'm about to hyperventilate somebody rushes over to him, wrapping an arm around his shoulder, pulling him away to meet somebody else. He turns back, looks at me and winks. My pussy sparks inside my knickers. My head tells me I don't know this man, not really – but my pussy doesn't give a fuck. If I had the chance, I would take it.

I start dancing again, hoping against hope he'll come back, enjoying the way my body moves more than ever after his compliment. But he doesn't return and, looking around the room for him, I can't see him anywhere. I go looking for the bathroom, telling myself on the way how unreal tonight has been – if he's left already then it doesn't matter: I met him, I spoke to him, I even *flirted* with him.

But as it turns out, my luck hasn't run out just yet . . .

I open a door to what I think is the loo, but find I'm in a dressing room instead. There's a long sofa, chairs in front of backlit mirrors, tables of flowers and fruit baskets – and in front of me, in an en suite with the door open, is a walk-in shower, a huge square shower head raining water down on to . . . *him* – the genius of my dreams. He's facing me, lathering himself up with soap, and he's completely naked, his cock hanging between his legs. My mouth falls open.

He laughs. He bends his knees and tips his head back, like he did on stage earlier, then says loudly over the running water, 'I can't believe it – I was literally just thinking about you.' When I don't say anything –

because I *can't* say anything – he says, 'You better come closer.'

I swallow. 'Why?' I manage.

He tilts his head to one side. With a cheeky smile he says, 'So I can check you're not a mirage.'

I close the door behind me with a click. I walk slowly towards him. He switches off the shower, the last of the soap suds dripping off his body. I walk on to the sopping tiles of the shower floor. And then I stop an inch away from him because I'm not sure where to start – it's not every day you're in an actual real-life dream.

'You've only just met me,' he breathes, his beautiful eyes travelling over my lips. 'Are you sure you want to do this?'

I look down at his cock. It's getting aroused before my eyes, springing more and more upright. It has a curve to it, a freckle on one side. *I'm looking at his cock*, I think. *His actual cock.*

'I *definitely* want to do this,' I say. The magic words. He puts his hands on either side of my face and kisses me hungrily, slipping his tongue into my mouth. I wrap my arms around his neck, feeling his now hard cock against my groin. The water on his body soaks through my clothes on to my skin. He pushes me up against the wet tiled wall and I run my hands through his soaking hair and across his smooth back. I'm highly aware of my pussy, hot and swelling between my legs.

He picks me up and I wrap my legs around him. I feel light as a feather in his arms – of course he's strong; he has to work out like hell to keep his stamina up through his tours. He walks me out of the shower and back into the dressing room, still kissing me deeply, and lays me down on the sofa. I kick off my shoes, reach down and undo my jeans button and push them down over my hips. He pulls them off me as I take off my top, fling away my bra. He lowers his weight on to me and the heaviness of his wet body against mine feels divine. I wrap my legs around him again. He kisses my neck, long, lingering, wet kisses, and arches his back, rubbing his hard cock rhythmically against my pussy trapped inside my knickers, the feel of the friction enticingly frustrating. His skin is still hot from the shower and I cling on to him, grateful for his solidness, that he's not a figment of my imagination.

He sits up suddenly and swiftly pulls off and discards my knickers. While he goes to get a condom I sit up against the sofa, open my legs wide and start touching myself because if I don't I'm going to explode. I'm gloriously wet and I draw it around the whole of my pussy, over my hardening clitoris and my wanting lips.

He watches me as he walks back over, rolling the condom down the shaft of his cock. He says, with awe in his voice, 'You're so sexy.' The thrill of his praise makes me stand up and push him on to the sofa. I straddle him. Ever so slowly, I slide myself down on to him, every millimetre of my pussy enjoying the thick shaft of his penis, every nerve ending shuddering with delight. He has filled me up and it feels so incredible I don't know whether to laugh or moan. I rock back and forth on his hips, thrusting him deep into me. He takes my breasts in his hands and pushes them roughly together, then takes one of my nipples into his mouth and sucks on it, looking up at me with eyes I know so well. I tighten myself around his cock and he lets go of my nipple to groan with pleasure. I move quicker and bounce up and down, looking down at the man I've fancied for so long. The curve of his cock is angled perfectly to hit my G-spot and the pleasure is increasingly intense.

I lean forwards and take his chin in one of my hands. 'I want you to cum in my mouth,' I say without stopping my bouncing. He nods at me, his eyes wide and wanting. **I keep going, his cock sliding in and out of me, the pleasure building within me. I grip on to his shoulders, I tip my head back, I let out a long, gasping moan as I climax.**

He puts his hands under my armpits and lifts me off, throwing me on to the sofa. He throws away the condom, and stands over me with his beautiful, smooth, hard cock in my face. He beats himself and I open my mouth hungrily, expectantly, my pussy still throbbing from the orgasm.

'I'm going to cum,' he says. His eyes roll to the back of his head and my mouth is filled with his salty, sweet ejaculation. I have always wanted to swallow this man's cum. And now I have it, dribbling down my face, spilling over my tongue.

He crumples on to the sofa next to me while I lie my head back against the cushion, wiping my mouth. I close my eyes and wonder if I've just had one of the most memorable moments of my life. Then I look around me. On one of the tables by the backlit mirrors is what I want: a pad and pen. Feeling pretty tired, I force myself off the sofa to fetch it. Still vaguely out of breath, I hand them to him. He looks, confused, up at me, 'What's this for?'

'Your autograph.' I grin down at him. 'Please can you make it out to my friend Isla?'

AFTERCARE

It has been my pleasure, and hopefully yours too, to help you on this journey to connect with your body in such an intimate way. This book isn't just about how to masturbate – it's about giving yourself what you deserve, returning home in your body, and recognising, accepting and celebrating the pleasures that nature has made available to us.

I honestly believe that pleasure is just the start of this journey. Talking about sex, whether that's solo or otherwise, is an impactful and important conversation. It helps us be more confident and more connected with ourselves and others around us. I hope that's what you take forward from this book: the ability to articulate what you like and an ability to talk more openly about sex with your friends and family, as well as any partners you may have. More than anything I hope that any shame you might have felt about masturbating, or your desires or fantasies, will be left behind for ever.

Thank you for picking up this book and being curious to discover more. I can't wait to hear about what you unlock – come tell me on Instagram @florencebark. Remember that you deserve to feel this pleasure, and this journey of self-love is entirely your own, so carve it out in whatever way feels right to you. You've got this!

Peace, love and happy masturbating!

Florence x

BUILD YOUR OWN SEXUAL FANTASIES

Some people say there's a book in everyone – I like to say there's an erotic story in everyone! If you'd like to imagine your own unique fantasy but you're struggling to focus in on what would turn you on most today, I've compiled some thought starters for you over the next few pages. Read through each section and pick one (or three, or ten – whatever you like!) from the list, then see if from that you can create a sexy storyline to imagine while touching yourself. I'd love to hear from you if you do this – come on over to my DMs.

FANTASY NO.1

	+		+	
Location		Personality		Sexy stuff

FANTASY NO.2

	+		+	
Location		Personality		Sexy stuff

FANTASY NO.3

	+		+	
Location		Personality		Sexy stuff

LOCATIONS

Kitchen • Bedroom • Living room • Bathroom • Garden • Gym • Closet • Library • Cinema • Swimming pool • Sauna • Jacuzzi • Office • Supermarket • Changing room • Treehouse • Shed • Park • Field • Meadow • Theme Park • Hotel • Igloo • Lift • Lobby • Train • Plane • Car • Truck/lorry • Tractor • Restaurant • Limo • Garden centre • Shopping mall • Car park • Doctors' surgery • Police station • Dentists' surgery • Sporting pitch/arena

PERSONALITY OF PARTNER(S)

Cheeky • Naughty • Filthy • Angry • Cheerful • Loving • Romantic • Seductive • Sexy • Mean • Generous • Powerful • Submissive • Obedient • Moody • Excitable • Active • Outdoorsy • Frantic • Shy • Confident • Serious • Silly • Prudish • Sexual • Good • Evil • Frightening • Familiar • Comforting • Generous • Bossy • Laid-back • Flirty • Brooding • Unreadable • Aloof • Fun • Funny • Intelligent

SEXY STUFF

Breast play • Thumb/finger sucking • Hand job • Blow job • Fingering • Clit play • Cunnilingus • Dildo • Vibrator • Other sex toy not mentioned here • Teasing • Tickling • Tender sex • Ice cubes • Candle wax • Passionate sex • Rough sex • Bondage • Massaging • Stroking • Hair pulling • Tender kissing • Passionate kissing • No kissing • Choking • Spanking/whipping • Butt play • Anal • Threesome • Orgy • Voyeurism • Getting caught • Edging • Missionary • Girl on top • Reverse cowgirl • Standing sex • Sex from behind • Sex sitting on furniture • Spooning sex • Other position not mentioned here

ENDNOTES

1   https://www.glamourmagazine.co.uk/article/glamour-masturbation-survey

2   https://yougov.co.uk/topics/society/articles-reports/2022/02/10/orgasm-gap-61-men-only-30-women-say-they-orgasm-ev

3   https://www.psychologytoday.com/gb/blog/stress-and-sex/201510/the-orgasm-gap-simple-truth-sexual-solutions

4   Kerner, Ian, *She Comes First* (New York: William Morrow & Co, 2004)

5   Puppo, V. and Puppo, G. (2015), *Anatomy of sex: Revision of the new anatomical terms used for the clitoris and the female orgasm by sexologists*, Clin. Anat., 28: 293–304.

ACKNOWLEDGEMENTS

In having to write this section it is just dawning on me that I've written a published book! I've seen and read so many of these in my favourite authors works it feels so deeply gratifying to be writing my own. So to you, reader, thank you for bravely, courageously, lovingly buying and reading my book on a topic that isn't always easy to get involved in. It is people like you that make change happen. Keep being curious.

Thank you to my wonderful, supportive and talented editor Emily Barrett, who helped create the magic between these pages. I basically tortured her by making her read and edit erotic stories while in the office – even though she blushed through the chapters – and this book wouldn't exist without her. What a woman!

Thank you to my hero, my mother, who has been my number one fan since the day I was born. That didn't change when I started talking about sex for a living. I'm grateful to her every day for never saying a negative word, even when I broadcast all my very best blow job tips across the world (3.7 million views and counting) and even when I told her I needed a lift to a sex workers' rights protest in LA while we were on holiday – not only did she drive me there, she stayed and walked with us along Hollywood Boulevard with a huge grin on her face.

Thank you to my intern, Emm Cheeky, who sat with me while I wrote some of these erotic meditations, who went through all the tips with me to make sure they were the very best, and read the stories back to me so I knew they would sound okay in the audiobook. Your enthusiasm around all of these topics inspires me every time we work together!

And lastly, but definitely not least, thank you to my partner in crime, Reed Amber. If I had never met you, this book wouldn't have been written. You changed my life in the most crazy and best way possible. We created a huge change in the sex and relationship content space and have helped so many people. Our extremely lovely Curious F**kers – your support is everything. Reed is the Yin to my Yang, a true sister from another mister.

And in the words of Snoop Dogg, thank you to me for turning up every day to make this a reality. I've been learning to appreciate myself more – I hope this inspires you to thank yourself too. Even if it's just for buying a book that changed your masturbation game forever.